To my rock, my partner, my love, Will. Your unwavering support fueled every page, your keen edits sharpened the story, and your unwavering belief kept me going. This book, like everything we create together, is a testament to our incredible journey.

To my late father, whose love of learning continues to guide me. Thank you for teaching me to embrace every day with kindness. To my mother, a testament to resilience and strength, your work ethic is an endless source of inspiration to me.

And to my dearest children (my whole world), Sarah, Jude, Jonah, Lucas & Noah, this book is yours. May it whisper tales of possibility, ignite your dreams, and inspire you to chase after the big things in life. Remember, there's magic within you, just waiting to be written.

This book is for all of you. <3

THE ULTIMATE GUIDE TO BECOMING A

MEDICAL SCIENCE LIAISON

MSL

SUZANNE SOLIMAN

PHARMD, BCMAS

Copyright © Suzanne Soliman, 2024
Edited by: Global Bookshelves International, LLC
Designed by: Publishing in Doses, LLC
ISBN: 979-8-9907090-0-3
Printed in the United States of America.

https://www.drsuzannesoliman.com/

To comment on this book, send an email
to the author at suzy@drsuzannesoliman.com.

Notice
The author has made every effort to ensure the accuracy and completeness
of the information presented in this book. However, the author cannot be held
responsible for the continued currency of the information, any inadvertent
errors, or the application of this information to practice. Therefore, the author
shall have no liability to any person or entity with regard to claims, loss,
or damage caused or alleged to be caused, directly or indirectly, by the use
of the information contained herein.

Table of Contents

Foreword

It is with immense pleasure that I introduce you to this informative guide penned by the esteemed Dr. Suzanne Soliman, a true expert in the world of Medical Science Liaisons (MSLs). As someone who has dedicated years to navigating, changing and leading the evolving landscape of MSL careers, I can confidently say this book will prepare anyone aspiring to join this impactful field.

Dr. Soliman's expertise shines through every page. Her insights aren't just theoretical; they're forged from real-world experience, successes, and the challenges she personally overcame. This book isn't simply a how-to manual; it's a mentorship program distilled into chapters, offering invaluable guidance on:

- **Cracking the code:** Demystifying the MSL role, its diverse career paths, and the unique skill set it demands.

- **Building your fortress:** Equipping you with the knowledge and tools to excel in every aspect, from scientific expertise to communication mastery.

- **Networking like a pro:** Navigating the complex healthcare landscape and forging meaningful relationships with key stakeholders.

- **Advocacy alchemy:** Mastering the art of effectively communicating scientific data and advocating for better patient outcomes.

Dr. Soliman goes beyond the technical skill set needed to be an MSL. She infuses her wisdom with warmth, humor, and real-life anecdotes, making the journey relatable and engaging. You will feel her passion for the MSL profession radiate through the pages, inspiring you to embrace the challenges and revel in the rewards. Whether you're a student yearning to chart your MSL path, a seasoned professional seeking to refine your skills, or simply someone curious about this integral role within Medical Affairs, this book is your compass. It's a treasure trove of knowledge, practical advice, and encouragement, all delivered by a leader who truly understands the MSL journey. So, take the first step and turn the page and embark on your MSL adventure with Dr. Suzanne Soliman as your guide. Remember, the world of medical science needs your passion, expertise, and dedication. Let this book be your torch, illuminating the path to a fulfilling and impactful career as an MSL.

With fervent support,

Leona Blustein, PharmD, BCMAS, MBA
National MSL Leader

Preface

As someone deeply entrenched in the pharmacy profession, I have had the privilege of supporting thousands of professionals aiming to carve a path in the pharmaceutical industry. Throughout my multifaceted career as a pharmacist educator, pharmaceutical industry expert, and hiring manager, I have encountered a recurring theme across the CVs I have reviewed and interviews I have conducted. Many individuals tend to overlook seemingly minor details that could set them apart in their career trajectories: verbal and written communication skills! This oversight is particularly apparent among prospective Medical Science Liaison (MSL) candidates, despite their impressive academic backgrounds and degrees like an MD, PharmD, or PhD.

Furthermore, candidates receive little to no guidance on industry positions during their academic training. For example, a study by Marshall University School of Pharmacy showed that 88% of students initially lacked substantial knowledge about the pharmaceutical industry as a career option.[1] Another study by the Accreditation Council for Medical Affairs (ACMA) highlighted that 73% of pharmacy graduates felt that their schools did not adequately prepare them for a job in the pharmaceutical industry.[2]

I want to help change these statistics. This book aims to help you land that coveted MSL role, whether it's your first role or fifth. In providing a step-by-step approach, my book will guide you on how to stand out and secure your dream position. *The Ultimate Guide to Becoming a Medical Science Liaison (MSL)* is about how to create a favorable image with employers. I offer insights on crafting a compelling Curriculum Vitae (CV) and coach you on the steps needed to ace your interviews. Although other books out there may provide similar guidance, this book is explicitly aimed at professionals who are aspiring Medical Science Liaisons—those entering the profession, seeking an initial position, changing their position, looking to power their career, switching career paths, or returning to the field after a hiatus

Who am I to offer advice?

Hi! Please allow me to introduce myself. My name is Suzy, and while my training is in pharmacy, I have always felt the urge to do "more" beyond traditional pharmacy. I distinctly remember sitting in my therapeutics class as a second-year pharmacy student at the University of Illinois at Chicago College of Pharmacy. I realized then that the role of a pharmacist would change in the next 20 years, and my career trajectory since then has been anything but linear. At the age of 26, I landed my first MSL role in cardiology. Here's how it happened: after graduation, I completed my primary care pharmacy residency and ventured into academia as a cardiology faculty member at Midwestern University Chicago College of Pharmacy. Following a research presentation at a clinical meeting in cardiology, I was approached by a recruiter for an MSL position. After a successful interview, I landed that job! Over the next few years, I worked in-house in pharma, where I developed assessment tools for my MSL team, which was comprised of physicians, pharmacists, PhDs, and nurses. My career then took me back to academia as an Assistant Dean of Academic Affairs at the University of Illinois at Chicago. After relocating to the East Coast, I assumed the role of Associate Dean at Touro College of Pharmacy in New York before returning to the industry as a Chief Medical Officer of the Accreditation Council for Medical Affairs (ACMA). I currently hold numerous faculty appointments at esteemed institutions, including the University of Illinois Chicago College of Pharmacy, Rutgers School of Pharmacy, St. John's College of Pharmacy and Health Sciences, and Fairleigh Dickinson School of Pharmacy and Health Sciences.

During the social media boom, I took to social media to answer career-related questions. I quickly garnered over 400,000 followers, and I immediately realized there was an information void among job seekers in the pharmaceutical industry. And that is why I decided to write this book! Drawing on my successes guiding and mentoring thousands of students "breaking into" the industry, I want to share insider insights and empower you on your career journey by demystifying what it takes to land that coveted MSL position. Embedded throughout this book you will find additional insider truth tips from me that I hope will guide you along the way.

Did you know that **80% of pharmacists** who currently work in pharma did not undergo a fellowship?[2] Whether you completed a fellowship or not, there are ways to open doors for you in this industry, and I am about to spill the secrets.

History of the Medical Science Liaison (MSL) Position

● — ● — ● →

To attain the role of a Medical Science Liaison (MSL), we need to visit the nuanced backstory that has shaped MSLs into the esteemed professionals they are today. Let's peek into the historical roots and evolution of this role within the medical landscape.

The Changing Landscape in Life Sciences

Today's life sciences industry is witnessing a paradigm shift: the traditional sales force in the pharmaceutical industry is declining while field MSL roles continue to rise. This shift was fueled by the growing complexity of healthcare, the ever-expanding therapeutic areas, and the need for timely and accurate information. With breakthroughs in areas like biologics and immunotherapy, personalized medicine, pharmacogenomics, artificial intelligence, digital health, and rare or orphan disease products, the boundaries of what is possible in healthcare are constantly expanding! This is evident not only in developing novel therapies but also in understanding diseases at a molecular level. As a result, the industry has been repositioning itself towards more collaborative approaches to provide specialized knowledge on the latest data and therapeutic options to Healthcare Providers (HCPs). This is precisely where MSLs come in. As a pivotal part of the Medical Affairs team, they act as scientific partners for healthcare stakeholders, effectively connecting clinical development with commercial success by fostering communication.

According to research presented at the American Society of Health-System Pharmacists (ASHP), medical science liaisons have been on the rise since 2005, while pharmaceutical sales representatives have been declining. The Accreditation Council for Medical Affairs (ACMA) reports that the number of MSL positions has increased by more than 300% in the previous decade alone.[3] This growth is also driven by the increasingly stringent regulatory and compliance requirements and high competitiveness in the industry, with pharma/biotech companies continuously focusing on extending their product portfolio to grab the market.

From Pharmaceutical Sales Representatives (PSRs) to MSLs: A Greater Emphasis on Scientific Expertise

The first Medical Science Liaisons were established by the pharmaceutical company Upjohn (acquired by Pfizer) in 1967.[4] The medication that caused the MSL rise was tolbutamide (Orinase®). It was introduced as an oral medication for treating Type 2

Diabetes (T2D) at a time when insulin injections were the only available treatment, sparking interest among healthcare providers for information about Orinase. Upjohn saw a need to have specially trained staff to operate in the field and provide scientific and clinical information to physicians.

The first MSLs were experienced sales representatives who also possessed a scientific background and high social skills. However, as the demands and regulations evolved, so did their roles. These new professionals no longer wanted to retail products but to serve as resources of scientific expertise. In the early 2000s, several companies began disbanding their current MSL teams for professionals with clinical and/or scientific training. The MSL movement grew as more specialty drugs were approved by the FDA, increasing the need for advanced clinical and scientific professionals to educate HCPs. In the early 2000s, however, companies began requiring advanced degrees such as PharmD, MD, or PhD to take the MSL role. Research today via a recent benchmark study demonstrates that more than 90% of current MSLs have a terminal degree.[5]

For decades, pharmaceutical companies relied solely on Pharmaceutical Sales Representatives (PSRs) to disseminate information on their products.[6] For the vast majority, PSRs generally have little to no background in science but instead rely on their sales prowess to market their products to medical professionals and, thus, to the public. In contrast, MSLs bring scientific expertise to the table, with most having specialization in their respective fields.

In 1995, there were about 38,000 PSRs employed, and their number grew to approximately 102,000 in 2005. However, after that, PSR employment saw a downward trend, reaching just 68,400 in 2017. On the other hand, in 2004, there were about 5,000 MSLs nationwide. Between 2005 and 2015, the number of MSLs employed increased from approximately 10,000 to 40,000. Today, globally, more than 210,000 MSLs are employed, a remarkable **increase of 525%**! According to the United States Bureau of Labor Statistics, employment for MSLs is projected to grow 17% from 2021 to 2031, a rate greater than the average growth of all the other occupations.[7]

PSRs and MSLs Change Over Time

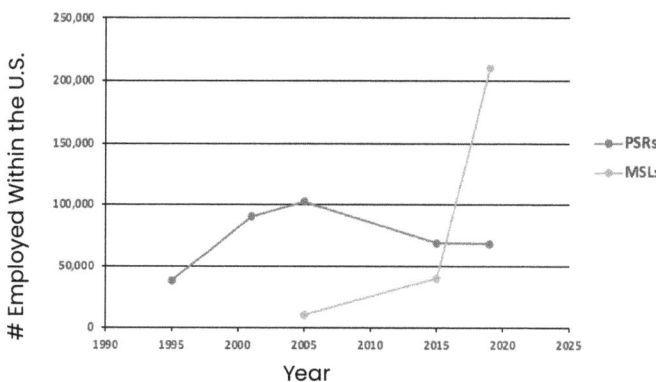

Figure 1: Shifts in MSL Employment Trends

PSRs and MSLs Change Over Ten Years

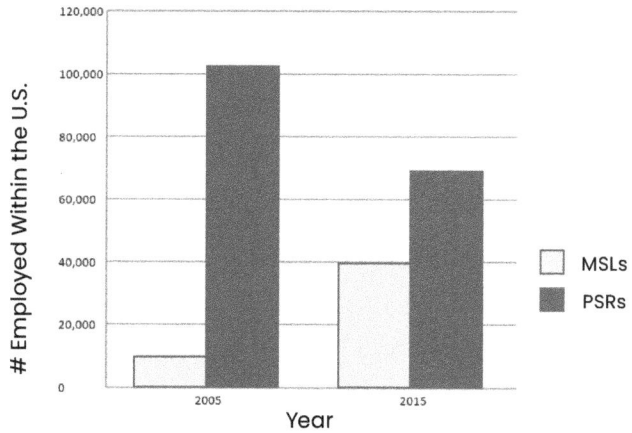

Figure 2: A Ten-Year Comparison of PSR and MSL Employment

According to several studies, a major reason behind the growth is that Healthcare Providers (HCPs) trust and rely on information from other "peer-like" colleagues—individuals with advanced degrees and training like MD, PharmD, and PhD. An ACMA analysis revealed that among MSLs, 40% hold PharmD degrees, 27% hold PhDs, and 30% hold MDs. At the same time, the remaining are Nurse Practitioners (NPs), Physician Assistants (PAs), and Doctors of Osteopathy (DO).[8] While the majority of MSLs have primary degrees of PharmD, MD, or PhD in the life or physical sciences, other careers, such as Nurse Practitioners, Doctors of Osteopathy, Physician Assistants, or other medical professionals, may hold an MSL position.[9]

HCPs often supplement their training on changes in available treatments when they interact with field representatives from life science companies. They rely heavily on MSLs for product and literature updates. In fact, MSLs may spend around an hour interacting with physicians through presentations. In contrast, the average time PSRs spend with physicians is just under two minutes. Because MSLs have specialized education, they can reactively cover a broader range of topics in their discussions than a sales executive, including data emerging from congresses, ongoing studies, research that has been published or abstracts presented, and competitor products. MSLs must adhere to specific policy stipulations regarding proactive or reactive discussions. Still, some of those policies differ from company to company. Strict regulatory guidelines dictate what MSLs can and cannot discuss.

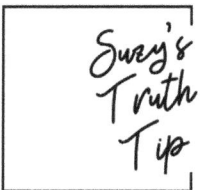

While both Pharmaceutical Sales Representatives and Medical Science Liaisons work within the pharmaceutical industry, their roles differ significantly in terms of their focus, responsibilities, and objectives. PSRs concentrate on promoting and selling products, whereas MSLs are the scientific link in the puzzle and focus on scientific exchange, education, and relationship-building with healthcare professionals.

Additionally, MSL success metrics are not based on the number of prescriptions written. It would be inappropriate for MSLs to learn about the prescribing habits of a provider, given that MSLs are scientific communicators. Companies have policies against using MSLs to determine prescribing behavior.

In 2018, the world was overtaken by the "opioid crisis." This put many pharmaceutical companies, like Purdue, who pushed the PSRs to boost OxyContin prescriptions, at the heart of a firestorm.[10] In response, many companies shifted towards employing MSLs, laying off the sales representatives for more impartial education, aiming to mitigate risk and ensure informed decision-making.

Physicians are not the only external stakeholders in the industry. The influence of external stakeholders has expanded significantly. Payers, Pharmacy Benefit Managers (PBMs), regulatory Key Opinion Leaders (KOLs), and patient advocacy groups, to name a few, provide insights to the pharma industry about trends in the healthcare landscape.

Access to healthcare providers is more challenging than ever. Physician reimbursement has decreased, causing HCPs to prioritize their time to see more patients and deal with more administrative hurdles. They value their time and are more apt to share it with MSLs than with commercial field forces.

On the other hand, a thorough understanding of our complex health system, such as Integrated Delivery Systems (IDNs) and Accountable Care Organizations (ACOs), is needed, as is a strong understanding of cross-functional groups in pharma. With regulatory requirements, ethical standards, and compliance becoming more stringent, companies are finding themselves in need of specialists to help them navigate through heightened scrutiny from regulators. Today, MSLs are integral to the medical department, operating independently of commercial functions.

Understanding the MSL Role

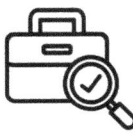

Before jumping into a position or doing a job search, you should make sure your personality and values align with the job you seek! If you have a passion for both science and communication, a career as a Medical Science Liaison (MSL) may be the perfect fit. When you consider the communication skills you have demonstrated in the past, think about whether you delivered any formal presentations, met with Key Opinion Leaders (KOLs), networked at conferences, or even sent simple emails to groups. All of that could contribute to your communication skills experience! An MSL should also be a captivating speaker, a good listener, and an effective communicator. Finally, MSLs must have excellent networking skills and be able to build and maintain relationships with healthcare professionals to establish credibility and trust.

How to Know if the MSL Role is Right for You

If your goal is to break into an MSL role, there are several questions you should consider asking yourself:

1. Am I willing to relocate if needed? Am I willing to travel?

2. What skills do I currently have that I'll need for the job I want?

3. Are there ways I can gain more experience now to make myself a more viable candidate in the future?

4. Am I willing to take another non-MSL position within a pharmaceutical company or consulting company/vendor to eventually progress to the MSL role?

There are certainly more questions to ask. Still, these questions provide an excellent starting point for clarifying what you're willing to do upfront.

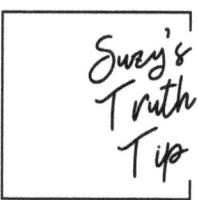

When reflecting on the travel and relocation question, really think about your life and how much time you can be away from home! The way MSLs conduct their jobs requires travel, primarily if the role covers multiple states. You'll travel to appointments, home offices for internal meetings, and conferences across the nation.

MSL Roles and Responsibilities

Very few people comprehend the role, responsibilities, and duties of the Medical Science Liaison, and it's fascinating to note that the MSL's responsibilities vary significantly from company to company. MSLs may be responsible for a wide range of activities, including:

- Educating healthcare providers about new medications

- Providing support to healthcare providers and patients

- Collecting data on the use of medications

- Conducting market research

- Developing marketing materials

- Ensuring that patients have access to the information and support they need to manage their chronic diseases

MSLs usually focus on a specific therapeutic area or disease state (e.g., oncology, rare disease, cardiology, endocrinology, infectious disease, hematology, rheumatology, etc.). These MSL roles can end up working for a biotechnology, medical division, pharmaceutical, clinical research, or managed care organization. The MSLs serve as scientific or disease state experts and are primarily responsible for establishing, cultivating, and fostering collaborative relationships between thought leaders and the companies they represent. In the majority of organizations, the MSL reports to the Medical Affairs Department. They provide these stakeholders with access to the latest scientific data and clinical evidence on their company's products, as well as insights into the company's research and development pipeline. MSLs also play a key role in gathering feedback and insights from HCPs on the company's products and services to take back to their company, which can then ultimately shape the overall strategy of their product.

Depending on the strategies and business objectives of the medical company, MSLs may have the following responsibilities:[11]

- During the early drug development phase, MSLs work on generating interest among external experts in the scientific aspects of new molecules and their mechanisms of action. They may also interact with the clinical development program through clinical trial site interactions.

- During the pre-launch phase, MSLs provide in-depth scientific insights about the drug to the KOLs, raise awareness, lay the groundwork for market access, and launch and present data at scientific meetings.

- During the launching of the product, MSLs focus on educating stakeholders about the clinical evidence and how to use the drug within clinical practice, aligning their activities with the overall commercial plan to support the product's success in the market.

- After the product has been launched, a large part of the role of MSLs is to address prescribers' inquiries along with continued medical education and implementation of publication- and investigator-initiated study plans. Another important MSL activity is to help determine the product strategy and implement the operational plan for real-world data generation.

Throughout all these stages, medical science liaisons (MSLs) play a crucial role in ensuring that internal stakeholders stay informed with the most recent clinical data and knowledge about therapy and the disease area.

MSL Career Progress

The titles of MSLs, including medical liaisons, medical managers, regional scientific managers, clinical liaisons, and scientific affairs managers, may vary depending on the company.

Typically, the career trajectory for an MSL may replicate the following order:

Senior MSL > MSL Manager > Senior Medical Director

More senior roles are typically located at the company's headquarters and involve more strategic work. The following list shares insights into the advanced roles of next step careers of an MSL.[12]

Senior Medical Science Liaison

Senior MSLs have honed their expertise to become authorities in their field, often overseeing larger territories. They frequently engage with KOLs and directly address the needs of healthcare professionals. Their tasks involve gathering insights from the medical community, identifying treatment gaps, and addressing challenges. Senior MSLs regularly update management on progress and hurdles, ensuring adherence to protocols and policies.

Medical Science Liaison Manager

The next step to climb is that of a medical science liaison manager. It is also a possible starting point for physicians wanting to move into medical affairs. MSL Managers oversee teams of MSLs, ensuring that they are up-to-date in their assigned therapeutic area and are aligned with the company's brand and medical strategy. They are often the face of a company and will take responsibility for entire teams.

Medical Director

Climbing to the top of the ladder, we have the medical director role, also referred to as a senior medical director or executive director. Their role involves planning, executing, and overseeing the recruitment and promotion of staff. Medical directors also foster relationships with other directors to strengthen networks. It is not always easy to grow after becoming an MSL, so it is important to establish your name at the company so you can grow into these roles.

MSL Salary Insights

In the ever-changing landscape of medical affairs, the role of Medical Science Liaisons also continues to change—they continuously strive to adapt to new specialists and redefine how teams engage with key opinion leaders. Being one of the highest-paying non-executive positions in the industry, their salary reflects the exceptional value and expertise they bring to their employers and stakeholders. MSLs typically receive a base salary and a bonus, based on how well the company performed or sometimes based on how the product line that the MSL worked for performed.

Let's break down the salary figures for MSLs. On average, a Medical Science Liaison can expect to earn around $176,000, while a Senior MSL may command approximately $195,000. Moving up the ladder, MSL Managers typically receive higher compensation, with an average salary of $209,000. Those at the level of Director of Medical Affairs earn an impressive $232,000, while Vice Presidents of Medical Affairs top the chart with a substantial average salary of $324,000.[13] In addition to a competitive base salary, MSLs can expect an annual bonus between 15-30% of their base salary–usually based on their company's performance and individual performance. Many companies offer stock options as another form of compensation, notably occurring at biotech companies. For example, several years ago, Intercept Pharmaceuticals' stock price surged over 2000% in one day, making many MSLs wealthier overnight. With your dedication and commitment to honing your skills and performance, you can look forward to receiving significant annual salary increases. According to some sources, MSLs can expect an average salary increase of 8% to 12% over 5 years, depending on their performance, location, and industry.

MSLs often undergo assessment based on Key Performance Indicators (KPIs) that evaluate their interactions with healthcare professionals (HCPs), their ability to share scientific knowledge, and their skill in facilitating scientific discussions. These KPIs can be divided into Quantitative KPIs (the number of HCPs engaged and the number of presentations given) and Qualitative KPIs (level of satisfaction among HCPs, the impact of MSL interactions on HCP prescribing behavior, and the overall contribution to the company's medical affairs strategy). Both of the KPIs are considered when assessing performance for considerations of bonuses or promotions.

The following table shows the average salaries for field-based medical affairs professionals in the United States, based on data collected by the Accreditation Council for Medical Affairs and the ACMA Trends Report (2022).

Career Title	Average Annual Salary
MSL	$176K
Senior MSL	$196K
MSL Manager	$209K
MSL Director	$232k
VP of Medical Affairs	$324K

Does Therapeutic Area Influence MSL Salaries?

One of the surprising facts many newcomers to the pharmaceutical industry entering the MSL role realize is that salary range is closely tied to the therapeutic area you work in. For example, oncology or rare disease professionals tend to have a higher salary than infectious diseases. Much of this is driven by market dynamics and the evolution of various therapeutic areas as it relates to improvements in treatment options and types.

The following table shows the average salaries for MSLs in various therapeutic areas worldwide, according to data from the ACMA Trends Report (2022).

Therapeutic Area	Average Annual Salary
Oncology	$160K
Hematology	$155K
Gastroenterology	$148K
Immunology	$146K
Dermatology	$145K
Rare Diseases	$143K
Rheumatology	$142K
Psychiatry	$135K
Infectious Diseases	$134K
Nephrology	$132K
Cardiology	$125K
Autoimmune	$125K
Endocrinology & Metabolism	$125K
Neurology	$122K

Challenges and Opportunities

While an MSL role can be immensely fulfilling, it is important to prepare yourself for the challenges you may have to face as an MSL.

A big part of the job involves extensive travel. Even when you're not in the field, it's crucial to maintain communication with thought leaders from your home office. As healthcare continues to push into a more digital and virtual space, maintaining relationships with KOLs, HCPs, and internal stakeholders has become more challenging as well.

It is essential that MSLs stay up to date with current literature and evolving medical knowledge and technologies. Those with less clinical experience may find it a bit more challenging to understand health systems and keep up with advancements, but they should not feel discouraged. Instead, use this as an opportunity for personal and professional growth through active engagement in conferences, scientific exchanges, and pursuing advanced degrees or certifications. MSLs must also navigate complexities surrounding data privacy, transparency, and conflicts of interest while upholding their commitment to providing accurate, unbiased information.

Furthermore, because the industry has become highly competitive, with multiple companies offering similar products or therapies, MSLs play a crucial role in distinguishing strategies that set their products apart from the rest. An MSL must have exceptional time management skills, balancing multiple responsibilities, including responding to inquiries, conducting scientific presentations, and managing projects. As an MSL, you have the opportunity to impact patient care and establish yourself as a thought leader in a respective therapeutic area by contributing to scientific publications, presenting at conferences, and participating in advisory boards.

CHAPTER 3

Routes to an MSL Career

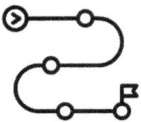

Embarking on a journey to find the right path toward an MSL career can often feel like navigating through a labyrinth without a clear map. Even with a significant rise in job opportunities within this field, the path remains ambiguous for many. This lack of clarity largely stems from the information gap that persists among students and job seekers. While networking is usually the most common way of discovering MSL opportunities, securing the role requires specific qualifications and strategic planning.

Much like different streams flowing into a river, there are diverse pathways that can lead you to become a Medical Science Liaison. These pathways may be generally categorized into the three routes. No matter where you begin, your educational background and training will guide you in choosing one of these three routes described in the table on the following page.

Route 1	Experienced Healthcare Professional or Experienced PhD → MSL
Route 2	Experienced in Various Areas of the Life Sciences or Pharmaceutical Industry → MSL
Route 3	Recent Graduate or Fellow → MSL

Most entry routes fall under the umbrella of the three routes mentioned above; however, there are ways to strengthen your candidacy. You are an expert in academia within a specialized field. For example, you have worked in cardiology your entire career by rounding with the team, teaching cardiology students and cultivating relationships with the best physicians. You have established yourself as an expert and can leverage your way into the industry. Experienced healthcare professionals who are interested in becoming an MSL should consider ways to showcase a level of expertise in a particular area and effectively market themselves to pursue Route 1. This route encompasses anyone who has worked and is experienced in their area such as someone who is a cardiologist and has dedicated their entire career to cardiology teaching cardiology students and cultivating relationships with the best physicians. You are already an expert in your area. If you are more of a generalist such as a community pharmacist, it is important to note that you are still an "expert." Find the area you have excelled in for example, you are an immunization or immunology expert and make that your part to stand out.

If you are currently working in managed care or managed-markets or in any area of the life sciences you can transition as an MSL. Many transition from medical information or working at a clinical research organization (CRO). This is all part of Route 2. You have demonstrated success in a non-clinical position and leverage that.

If you are a recent graduate or fellow, forming relationships and networking with your mentors/teachers and other industry professionals can help. Also, this demonstrates you have an interest in a specific area. These would be Route 3.

Whether you are working or not, as long as you have your degree, you can transition into the MSL field.

Suzy's
Truth
Tip

No license? No problem! There are plenty of reasons why someone may choose not to pursue professional licensure, but you will prevail and still be able to work in the industry without it. In fact, many who work in industry do not renew their licenses because, for a position as a Medical Science Liaison, it is often not needed.

Building Your Social Media Presence

In our previous chapters, we delved into the origins of Medical Science Liaisons and the various routes you can take toward your dream role. But in today's digital age, getting to that dream role begins with building your social media presence. It is no surprise that having a poor social media presence will significantly hinder you from landing the role you want.

Think about it: If you do not exist online, you do not exist. So, buckle up as we navigate the intricacies of building and maintaining your social media presence on your way to MSL success!

The Importance of Online Presence

Maintaining a professional and favorable online presence can significantly impact your job prospects in the pharmaceutical industry. Almost every company you interview for will search for your name online to learn more about you. Most pharmaceutical companies have a presence on at least one social media platform, and you should, too. According to a 2022 survey by Jobvite, 77% of employers use social media to screen candidates.[14] This includes Google, Facebook, LinkedIn, and X (formerly Twitter). The survey also found that 57% of employers have rejected a candidate based on information they found online.

Here are some of the reasons why employers use Google to search for potential candidates:

- **To verify the candidate's qualifications**: Employers want to make sure that the candidate has the skills and experience they are looking for. They may google the candidate's education, work experience, and certifications.

- **To get a sense of the candidate's personality**: Employers want to know if the candidate is a good fit for their company culture. They may look into the candidate's social media profiles to see what he/she/they are interested in and how that candidate interacts with others.

- **To find any red flags**: Employers also search the candidate's online profiles to determine if there is anything in his/her/their past that could disqualify that candidate from the job, such as criminal records, negative social media posts, or financial problems.

It's important to remember that employers are not looking for perfect candidates. They are seeking individuals who are a good fit for their company culture and have the potential to grow and develop.

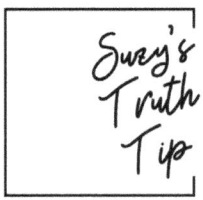

Take a moment to search for your full name on the internet. What does your online presence say about you? If you are concerned about your online footprint, take proactive measures to clean up your online presence and be mindful of what you post online. This will help you present yourself in the best light possible and increase your chances of landing a job.

Selecting the Right Social Media Platforms

When starting your social media presence, it is important to select the right social media platforms. Not all social media platforms are created equal. Some platforms are more popular with healthcare professionals than others.

For example, X (formerly known as Twitter) and LinkedIn are popular platforms for medical professionals to share news, research, and insights. On LinkedIn, you will find groups related to medical affairs. A group that I suggest for LinkedIn is "The Board Certified Medical Affairs Specialist (BCMAS) Network." A group I suggest on Facebook is the "Pharmacist Moms Pharmaceutical Industry." You can engage in discussions, share insights, and network with professionals in the field. You will also find profiles of companies sharing updates and job openings.

X is also a great platform where you can follow and engage with influential KOLs.

Networking apps like Sermo and Doximity cater specifically to HCPs, so it is easier to find and connect with thought leaders and medical groups to showcase your expertise.

While Facebook, Instagram, and TikTok are more popular for personal use, they can still be used to connect with potential KOLs and other healthcare professionals. There are Facebook groups focused on pharmaceuticals/biotech, medical affairs, and MSL careers. Participate in discussions, share relevant articles, and network with group members.

There are also specialized forums and websites you can explore, like Cafepharma, Inc. and BioSpace, which are dedicated to pharmaceutical and medical affairs professionals. These platforms regularly feature job listings, industry news, and networking opportunities through active message boards where you can engage and establish your presence.

Strategies for Building A Successful Social Media Presence

Not sure where to begin? LinkedIn is often a great place to start. Make sure your profile is complete by including a bio with a professional picture, work history, and recommendations. When reaching out to connect with others, always personalize your message to introduce yourself and build your network. Use industry-related keywords or keywords relevant to your niche and therapeutic expertise. You may also incorporate your knowledge of regulatory documents and clinical guidelines relevant to your therapeutic area.

Also, ensure that your LinkedIn profile is public and personalize your URL so that you are easy to find on the platform. Use a professional email address—your first name, last name, or initials are always best. For example mine is: https://www. linkedin.com/in/suzannerabi.

X is another way to build your online presence. It is a great way to follow companies and recruiters, share information, and find job opportunities. You can also find out what is important to the companies you are interested in. Try linking your X and LinkedIn accounts, and you may end up following similar people or companies. Consider using the same professional headshot across all professional platforms to help identify you, especially if you have a popular first and last name. If one platform has a photo of your pet dog, while another has you on top of a mountain with your dog, and another is of you in a business suit, it may be difficult to determine if they are following the right or same person. Also, do not use unprofessional photos such as you in a bathing suit or with a glass of wine.

Whether it is X or LinkedIn, the formula for building a successful social media presence remains the same:

+ *Find your niche.* Your niche includes your passions, skills, and values. It is important to demonstrate this during the interview and on your CV, resume, or application. When writing your cover letter and preparing for your interview, emphasize your area of expertise and your contribution to this focus. Highlight what sets you apart as a potential MSL.

✦ *Be authentic.* Authenticity is key to building genuine connections. If you can naturally show up and be yourself, your personality will be evident and shine through. Authenticity resonates with others, and they will be more eager to connect with you.

✦ *Share relevant content.* The key to building a successful social media presence is to share relevant content. This means sharing content that is interesting and informative to your target audience, i.e., KOLs, recruiters, human resources, etc. For a potential Medical Science Liaison, this could include news articles about your therapeutic area, research studies, or clinical trials. You could also share infographics, videos, or blog posts.

✦ *Be consistent.* The key to building a successful social media presence is to be consistent with your posting. This means posting new content regularly. The more you post, the more likely people are to see your content and engage with it.

✦ *Engage with your audience.* Simply sharing content and waiting for people to follow you may be an unrealistic expectation. You need to engage with your audience. This means liking, commenting, and retweeting content from other healthcare professionals. You can also start conversations by asking questions or sharing your thoughts and opinions. A great way to build an online presence and following is to engage with others and get "noticed." Imagine getting interviewed by someone that you have already conversed with on social media. The rule of 80/20 applies to posting on professional platforms. Approximately 80% of your posts should be professional posts related to the industry, and up to 20% can be tasteful personal life posts that provide insight into your life. This allows followers to feel like they can relate to you and know you have a healthy work/life balance and also that you are human and not AI-generated.

✦ *Keep in touch.* You'll find many of your mentors or even new connections are willing to help you. Do not hesitate to actively engage with their posts and keep in touch with them. I've had pharmacy students who completed a P4 rotation in medical affairs with me who reached out to me occasionally on social media (e.g., every 3, 6, or 12 months). Later on, I've even hired them. What stands out to me is their proactive approach—they take the initiative to stay connected, which is crucial. It shows they are invested in fostering ongoing relationships.

✦ *Use hashtags.* Hashtags are a great way to get your content seen by more people. When you use relevant hashtags, your content will show up in the search results for those hashtags. This means that more people will be able to see your content, even if they don't follow you. Using hashtags in the area you want to be recognized in is a great way to start. You can use hashtags like #medicalscienceliaison #medicalaffairs #oncology #cardiology #pharma #bcmas #msl #acma and more. You should also search these hashtags on all of the platforms and look for relevant content on these subjects.

These will help connect you with those people who are already discussing these topics.

✦ *Use analytics.* Most social media platforms offer analytics tools that can help you track your progress. These tools can show you how many people are seeing your content, who is engaging with it, and where your audience is located. This information can help you improve your social media strategy and reach more people.

Following these tips can help you build a solid social media presence as a prospective Medical Science Liaison. You can also create a robust online network. It is one of the most effective tools to research hiring managers or other key decision-makers before your interview. By sharing relevant content, engaging with your audience, and using the right hashtags, you can reach more people and make a positive impression on potential employers. You do not need to have a following of 100,000 to be relevant, but the goal is to exist online so that you are "trustworthy."

Identifying Key Opinion Leaders

Key Opinion Leaders (KOLs) are highly influential figures within the medical community. KOLs include experts, researchers, and physicians who are leaders in their fields. In the pharmaceutical and biotechnology sectors, KOLs play a crucial role as strategic allies, helping companies effectively accomplish their objectives.

While most companies have compiled a list of key KOLs, it's important to identify new ones continually. Tracking publications is a good way to identify potential KOLs. Leverage online platforms and databases such as PubMed to access pharmaceutical, clinical, and biomedical literature. Consider looking for publications and citation history by authors, keywords, journals, and more.

Events and conferences are, in my opinion, the most important source of KOL identification. Leaders in a specific field often take on roles as speakers, presenters, or session chairs. As a cardiovascular MSL, I monitored the American Heart Association events and followed those who presented critical information. I also paid attention to identifying emerging KOLs, who were often the up-and-coming fellows in specialized fields.

KOLs also have leadership roles on advisory boards and committees in national organizations like the American Heart Association or the American Society of Clinical Oncology, and they influence their respective domains, shaping industry trends and practices. Look into who is serving as an elective officer such as president or secretary of these professional organizations both locally and nationally. It will help determine who these KOLs are now and who is a rising star.

The Don'ts of Social Media

Always remember that hiring managers will check LinkedIn recommendations, and they will google to see who you are "online." Be careful what you post because it will stay there forever.

There have been cases of people losing their jobs over something they posted online. In contrast, many others have found themselves not getting hired after posting inappropriate content. Some individuals have been caught on camera for doing or saying something inappropriate or unlawful.

Your email address is often one of the first impressions you make in a professional setting. NEVER use unprofessional email addresses such as bigdog12345@hotmail.com or snoopygirl2222@aol.com, which may create a negative impression when a recruiter sees them.

Do not spam, stalk, or pester your contacts or potential employers. Do not argue about everything or topics that are controversial online. Your reputation matters. While sharing is encouraged, be mindful of oversharing. Recognizing and respecting the line between appropriate communication and invading someone's space is crucial.

Preparing the Curriculum Vitae

A Curriculum Vitae (CV) is like a detailed portrait of your professional and academic journey. When applying for jobs, your CV should not only capture your accomplishments but also showcase your potential as a standout MSL candidate. In this industry, where precision and thoroughness are paramount, your CV serves as the key to unlocking numerous opportunities. Let's delve into the art of crafting a compelling CV that will set you apart in the competitive landscape of MSL recruitment.

What is the objective of a CV?

A Curriculum Vitae (CV) is a comprehensive summary of your academic and professional history and is crucial when applying for jobs, fellowships, and other opportunities. A well-written CV can help you stand out from other candidates and increase your chances of securing the job or opportunity you want. Unlike a resume, which is a summary of the same information, a CV is more thorough and usually longer than one or two pages.

It is the preferred document for health professionals, academics, and people in other specialized professions, such as law, because it contains additional details about qualifications and activities. In contrast, a resume is used primarily when you are applying for a specific employment opportunity. A CV is the gold standard when applying for an MSL role.

What to Include in a CV

A CV normally begins with the words "Curriculum Vitae" at the top of the first page, followed by your contact information starting with your entire legal name or first name, middle initial, and last name. In parentheses, you can also specify a hyphenated name or your maiden name. Your personal information, such as your current, permanent, or temporary address, as well as your phone number and email address, should be listed. It could also contain your social media accounts like LinkedIn or X.

Education is typically the next section. This should include the schools you attended and the degrees you earned. When detailing your educational background, it's important to list them in reverse chronological order (start with the most recent and work backward). Always include the institution's name, location, the duration of your attendance, and the degree you earned.

Consistency is key. This ensures clarity and professionalism when presenting your educational journey. If you have an excellent academic record, it makes sense to highlight your achievements, such as grade point average, class rank, or graduation honors. However, it is best to remove everything high school-related because you already have a college degree. Avoid sharing personal information such as your birth date, the number of children you have, or your marital status. Similarly, unless specifically requested, refrain from including a headshot on your CV. This ensures a focus on your professional qualifications and avoids unnecessary distractions.

The third section should include your job titles, the companies you worked for, and your responsibilities. It should also include any relevant professional training you've undergone, such as residencies, fellowships, or certifications. You can list these in the educational section or create a separate section if there are a lot of them. Be sure to include the name and location of the training, the type of training received, the dates attended, and how long your certification is valid.

Your professional talents and abilities are the next most crucial area on your CV. This part should ideally be devoted to professional experience and should not include any unrelated work. People at the start of their careers, on the other hand, may prefer to mix professional and other work experiences under one section. Those with extensive work experience will want to exclude all other work experience. Volunteer experience can also be included in this section if your dedication was sustained over time and is relevant to your job application as an MSL. Oftentimes, potential employers view volunteer work equally as valuable as experiences gained through a paid opportunity. Additionally, volunteering within separate departments for public or community service is also something to include.

The next few sections are all relevant. You will want to add information on your licensure and/or certification. This will help you stand out, as many applicants are not licensed and/or certified in medical affairs. However, if you're not licensed, simply skip this section. Focus instead on showcasing your accomplishments and qualifications without mentioning that you were unable to pass your boards. If you are not certified, simply skip this section, but you should consider it. I will discuss this in a later chapter.

Your awards and honors can be in a separate section. Include anything you may have earned from college and beyond. There is a sample CV and template in this book to help provide some context on how to display this.

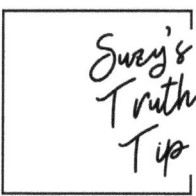

Move awards and honors to the top of your document right under your name if you have a lot of them. Remember, this is your chance to "brag!"

The research experience section is an excellent area to highlight any research and scholarly endeavors, including grants, collaborations, patents, and projects. Include the title, sponsoring agency or company, funding sought, submission date, and outcome. Additionally, list any publications in professional journals, authored books or reports, and relevant clinical presentations. You can also include any industry-related podcasts or events that you have been a guest or participant in.

Teaching experience holds significant weight in the profile of prospective MSLs. I would recommend dedicating a separate section to highlight your teaching experience and academic appointments. List the amount of hours you taught, the institution, the course number, the title, the dates, and the number of students. Additionally, mention your role as a mentor, precepting students, and preparing any course material. Teaching experiences should include all types of teaching experience and faculty appointments. Experiences you should include (but not limited to) are:

- Lecturing (virtual or in-person)
- Coordinating conferences
- Precepting students
- Precepting professionals
- Providing a continuing education course
- Giving workshops
- Teaching a recitation session
- Mentoring students or colleagues
- Writing a newsletter

Optimizing Your CV With Keywords

The digital age of recruiting is upon us, which means that all applicant tracking systems and recruitment websites have "search" functionality and even artificial intelligence tracking software, i.e., the Applicant Tracking Systems (ATS), which is designed to prescreen all candidates. As a result, corporate recruiters will run search queries based on specific keywords. If your CV lacks the required keywords for the job you are applying for, your information might never be found.

Over 97% of Fortune 500 companies use ATS, while 66% of large companies and 35% of small organizations also rely on them.[15] So, it's likely that the company you're applying to is using ATS as well. Using keywords that are relevant to the MSL position you're applying for in your CV will help you get noticed by potential employers and match the ATS specification. Upon submission, they'll look for specific job descriptions by keywords and will remove anyone the software deems as unqualified. So, keywords are critical to your success in getting a job.

As you edit your CV, think about which keywords a recruiter might use to find someone with your specific background.[16] Review job descriptions and similar job postings to see which common keywords are being used by prospective employers. Keywords can be job titles and descriptive words that relate to your job function. Make sure you also include a lot of information relevant to your therapeutic area.

Use a variety of keywords. Do not just use the same keywords over and over again. It is also important to use keywords that are specific to the company that you are applying to. For example, if you are applying for a job at a company that develops diabetes management drugs, you could use keywords like "diabetes," "insulin," and "GLP-1."

When using keywords, it is important to be strategic and integrate them throughout the CV. While you should incorporate keywords related to the job description, it is also important not to use keywords that are too common. Also, avoid keyword overstuffing, which is unnaturally forcing keywords to improve the search results, as this makes the CV appear unnatural.

Here are some additional tips for using keywords when searching for a Medical Science Liaison job:

- Use both broad and specific keywords. This will help you to reach a wider audience of potential employers.
- Use research or industry-specific keywords, including job titles, skills, certifications, and other relevant terms.
- Use keywords in your online profiles. This will help you be found by potential employers when they are searching for candidates.

By following these tips, you can use keywords to increase your chances of finding a Medical Science Liaison job.

Tips for Writing a CV

As a professor and mentor to thousands of pharmacists, I read and review resumes and CVs daily. I may not be a professional resume writer, but I do have a solid understanding of what a good resume or CV looks like. More importantly, I keep track of what is most effective and elicits the best response from potential employers. A well-written CV can help you stand out from the competition and achieve your career goals.

First, your CV is essentially your **brand on paper**. Make sure that all of the information you include on your resume works towards highlighting your niche and justifying your fit for the MSL role you seek.

Next, focus on the *style, formatting, and appearance* to enhance the overall impression of your CV. You can find professional templates online that will work well for your background and industry. You may ask to review your MSL friend's or colleague's CV to get some insights. The ideal font size is 12, but never go smaller than an 11-point font. Times New Roman, Arial, and Garamond are all good font choices. Always use dark text on a white background. Avoid excessive capitalization or underlining. Bold titles and ample white space can improve clarity and aesthetics.

It is always best to include a *Professional Summary* at the top of your CV. Think of it as a snapshot of your identity. This summary should outline your experience, skills, achievements, and areas of expertise. Remember, this is NOT your career objective. Write the summary in the third person to make it sound more professional.

Example of a Professional Summary:

A performance-driven Medical Affairs professional with over fifteen years of combined experience in healthcare, clinical research, and the medical industry, developing in-depth and productive relationships with key professionals in academic, clinical, and payor organizations to optimize business opportunities. Acknowledged for strong presentation, communication, and organizational skills to successfully direct complex projects among many levels of internal and external customers in multiple therapeutic areas, including Cardiovascular, Metabolic, and Nephrology. Currently seeking a field-based Medical Affairs role with a growing company.

Display your **contact information** prominently. Use the header option; your name should be bold with a larger font than the rest of the text. Add your credentials after your name, such as Ellie Smith, PharmD, CDE, or Ellie Smith, MD, PhD. List your titles correctly; begin with your highest degree, such as Jane Smith, PharmD, BCPS (NOT Jane Smith, BCPS, PharmD), followed by certifications, and finally, licenses if applicable. This confirms clarity and professionalism.

It is okay if you don't want to disclose your full address, but at least provide your base city. This helps potential employers understand your commuting distance or the potential territories you may cover as an MSL.

Your years of experience will dictate the **appropriate length** of your CV. Unlike resumes, which are typically one to two pages long, CVs can be longer as they thoroughly include publications, presentations, abstracts, journal articles, editorial tasks and reviews, awards, grant support, etc. However, the first two to three pages should capture the most relevant highlights of your career and experience.

If you have worked a long time for the same company (8-10 years or more), provide a comprehensive breakdown of the various roles and positions you held over that period. Feel free to **list each role separately,** along with the corresponding time frames.

When crafting your CV, **avoid using the pronouns "I" or "me."** While these pronouns are typically part of our everyday sentence structure, they become redundant in a professional CV.

Do NOT include irrelevant information such as political affiliation, religion, age, hobbies, and sexual preference. Additionally, it is not necessary to mention comments like

"Available to Interview" or "Can Start Immediately." Although it is very common, the statement "References Available Upon Request" can be left off as well. Employers will ask for references at the proper time regardless of whether they are offered via the resume.

Just like your social media presence, your CV should also *reflect your authenticity*. Make sure that you can back up all the claims you make and resist the urge to stretch the truth. You never know when your potential employer might fact-check you.

Prepare multiple versions of your CV. Customize it for each employer and/or role you are applying for so that you can highlight your background and skills for that specific role.

Your CV should *be free of all errors and typos*. You'll be surprised how many typos and spelling errors I find in the CVs of many applicants. Use spellcheck tools and thoroughly proofread your CV. You can also share it with your colleagues or family members, who can proofread it on your behalf.

Review and update your CV regularly. These revisions may include new responsibilities, achievements, training, promotions, special projects, or milestones, including publications, presentations, abstracts, journal articles, editorial tasks and reviews, awards, etc.

Do not forget to *update your LinkedIn profile* so that it is a mirror image of your final CV. Keep in mind that most recruiters and employers will cross reference your LinkedIn profile once they have your CV, so both must be a match.

You will also want to replace all weak action verbs and use replacements that are unique and powerful to highlight your accomplishments, not just list your job duties (since many job functions have similar duties).

Weak Verbs	Replacements
Assisted	Accelerated, Facilitated, Contributed
Collaborated	Partnered, Coordinated, Unified
Helped	Boosted, Enhanced, Cemented
Made	Engineered, Developed, Crafted
Organized	Orchestrated, Structured, Systemized
Responsible for	Oversaw, Managed, Administered
Tasked with	Headed, Planned, Produced
Supported	Bolstered, Sustained, Fortified

Your CV will earn you an interview, and your interview will earn you the MSL job! As a prospective MSL, your CV should include the following sections:

Information Type	Alternative Options
Education	Education and Training
	Education and Specialized Training
	Education and Postgraduate Training
Awards and Honors	Honors and Distinctions
	Selected Achievements
	Awards and Fellowships
	Academic Achievements
Licenses and Certificates	Professional Licensure
	Certificates
	Certifications
	Board Certification
	State Licensure

Academic Appointment	Teaching Experience
	Courses Taught
	Courses Developed
	Faculty Appointments
Experience	Internships
	Fellowships
	Residency
	Professional Experience
Publications	Recent Publications
	Select Publications
	Textbook Chapters
	Journal Articles
	Peer-reviewed Articles
	Poster Presentations
	Published Abstracts
Presentations	Invited Presentations
	Select Presentations
	Peer-reviewed Presentations
	Non-peer reviewed Presentations
	Invited Papers and Lectures
	Seminars Presented
Personal Interest	Hobbies
	Volunteer Experiences
References	Professional References

Here is a quick recap:

- Your CV should be formatted in a clear and concise way. Use a standard font, such as Times New Roman or Arial, and use a 12-point font size.

- Use white space to make your CV easy to read.

- Print your CV on quality paper, using a nice printer and avoid using wrinkled or torn paper.

- Before you submit your CV, be sure to proofread it carefully. Check for errors in grammar or spelling and ensure that it is free of typos.

- Do NOT include a career objective. Most healthcare professionals do NOT put one on their CVs. You may wish to include one; however, that can limit what position you may find.

- Be specific: When listing your work experience, be as specific as possible about your job titles, the companies you worked for, and your responsibilities. The more data, numbers, and dollar amounts you can mention, the better.

- Tailor your CV to the job: When you are applying for a job, be sure to tailor your CV to the specific position. Highlight the skills and experience that are most relevant to the job.

- Keep it concise: If you do not have a lot of experience, you can keep the CV brief and to the point.

- Update your CV regularly: Be sure to update your CV to reflect your latest accomplishments.

- When saving the document, save it as a PDF and use your full name as the file name. Do NOT have the document saved as a random number, word, etc. Using your name will make it easier to find and screen.

- Replace weak action verbs with replacements that can powerfully communicate your achievements.

A Proper CV Example

FIRST NAME, LAST NAME, DEGREE

City, State | Telephone # | Email | LinkedIn Profile

EXECUTIVE SUMMARY

Write this as a professional summary profile written in the third person. Alternatively, you can capture this in 4-5 bullets, if applicable.

PROFESSIONAL EXPERIENCE

ABC Company, New York, NY   **May 2018-Present**
Consultant

- 4-5 bullets focusing on accomplishments

Company XYZ, Greater New York City Area   **Sep 2016-May 2017**
Global/US Director, Business Development

- 4-5 bullets focusing on accomplishments

EDUCATION & CREDENTIALS

...

PROFESSIONAL ORGANIZATIONS

...

PUBLICATIONS

...

Curriculum Vitae Template

NAME: Mary Warren, PharmD, BCMAS
ADDRESS: 1234 S. Central Avenue
New York, New York 12345
PHONE NUMBER: 212-123-4567
Website or LinkedIn URL

Education

...

Honors and Awards

...

Professional Experience

...

Licenses

...

Publications

...

Presentations

...

Professional Memberships

...

Teaching Experience

...

Service Activities

...

References

Curriculum Vitae Example

John Smith, PharmD, BCMAS

Chicago VA Medical Center
100 VA Medical Center Drive
Chicago, IL 60606
Telephone: 111-111-1111
Facsimile: 222-222-2222
Email: johnsmith@gmail.com
Social Media: LinkedIn Profile URL

Education

Only include your GPA if you have a high GPA... and exclude otherwise.

**University of Kentucky
Medical Center**
Lexington, KY

PGY-2 Oncology Resident
2015–2016

Veterans Affairs Medical Center
Chicago, IL

PGY-1 Oncology Resident
2014–2015

**Chicago State University
College of Pharmacy**
Chicago, IL

Doctor of Pharmacy
2014

Loyola University Chicago
Chicago, IL

Pre-Pharmacy Curriculum
2008–2010

Awards & Recognition

Include this on top if this is relevant and you have something to show. If you do not, or if you have only one, then put it on the bottom.

Experience

University of Illinois at Chicago
Chicago, IL

**Clinical Pharmacist,
Oncology**
2016–Present

Walgreens Pharmacy
Chicago, IL

Pharmacy Technician
2008–2012

Pharmacy Practice Experience Rotations

These should only be included if you graduated less than five years ago or need fluff. If you already have a lot on your CV, do NOT put your rotations on your CV unless you did something relevant during your rotation.

Licenses & Certifications

Illinois State Board of Pharmacy	License #1234
CPR Certified, etc.	2024–present
BCMAS Certified	2018–present

Publications

...

Research Experience

Grants approved and funded
Patents

Presentations

Label this section as "selected presentations" if you have a lot of them. Differentiate if your presentation is peer-reviewed, invited, or just a general presentation.

Invited

Peer-reviewed

Non-peer reviewed

Invited Book Chapters

Professional Membership

Illinois Health-System Pharmacist Association

Recording Secretary	2016–2017
Vice-President	2017–2020

Chicago State University College of Pharmacy

Lambda Kappa Sigma, President	2013–2014
American Pharmacists Association, Secretary	2013–2014
Student Council Treasurer	2011–2012

Curriculum Vitae Example *(continued)*

Leadership Experience

List any leadership positions you have held since pharmacy school. It is important to note every position.

Service Activities

These are your volunteer activities, such as volunteering at your religious institution or local organizations.

National
Leukemia & Lymphoma Society Walkathon
Chairperson, Chicago, 2019

Local
Girl Scouts of America Troop Leader
Chicago, IL, 2020-Present

References

Available upon request

Note: you do not need to list this section for references unless requested.

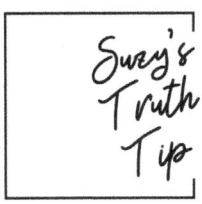

What are the best criteria in a competitive CV for an MSL?

- *Limited job jumps*
- *Consistency and loyalty in previous roles*
- *Current or recent MSL history*
- *Shadowing an MSL*
- *Strong experience in one or more therapeutic areas*
- *Having BCMAS certification*
- *Having a doctorate degree*
- *Having publications*
- *Good baseline knowledge*

CHAPTER 6

Crafting an Impactful Cover Letter

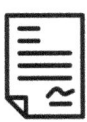

As you prepare to apply for your desired MSL position, it is important to remember the value of a well-written cover letter. With the right approach, your cover letter can be a crucial tool to securing the job of your dreams. In this chapter, we'll discuss the nitty-gritty of crafting a cover letter that's not just another document in the pile but rather the key to grabbing the attention of the recruiters.

What to Include in a Cover Letter

With so many applicants competing for a position and hiring managers having limited time, a cover letter should be clear and compelling, highlighting your most important attributes relating to the job. A 2023 survey found that hiring managers usually spend just 30 seconds to two minutes on a cover letter.[17] So, it's crucial to make your cover letter concise and impactful enough to grab their attention.

It is very likely that you will be e-mailing your resume to many companies or recruiters for consideration. Instead of having a cover letter as an attachment, consider incorporating a strong e-mail intro to act as a brief cover letter and resume highlight. This means your e-mail will only have one attachment (your CV/resume), which will ensure the reader will not have to open more than one document. To be safe, you can also include the full resume in the body of your e-mail (under the intro) in case the attachment is blocked by a spam filter.

Before you start writing, take the time to thoroughly research both the company and the particular role you're interested in. This background knowledge will help you customize your cover letter.

You should start with a *header/letterhead* where you input your name and contact information. *Greet* the hiring manager; try to find the name of the person reviewing applications for the job and address your letter to this person, e.g., "Dear Dr. Smith..."

The first sentence of the main body of the letter should *mention the job title* you are applying for and where you saw the posting for that role. After introducing yourself, *highlight your skills and achievements*. In the next part, explain how you are a good fit for the role and *the value you bring*. End the letter with a *professional signoff,* thanking the hiring manager for their time and consideration.

[Your Name]
[Your Address]
[City, State, ZIP Code]   } This should be your letterhead
[Your Email Address]
[Your Phone Number]

[Date]

[Company Name]
[Company Address]
[City, State, ZIP Code]

[Salutation]
[Body of Message]
[Signature]

Note: Use letterhead on top of the cover letter.

Suzanne Soliman, PharmD, BCMAS
1234 New Albany Street
New York, NY 10010
suzy@drsuzannesoliman.com
212-123-4567

September 1, 2024

Lisa Smith, MD, BCMAS
Pfizer
Medical Director

Dear Dr. Smith,
I am writing this in response to your recent notification regarding a vacancy for the post of Medical Science Liaison. I aspire to work as a medical scientific liaison in my career. For the last decade, I have acquired expertise in the field of oncology through my roles as a professor and clinician. I have also leveraged my experiences to cultivate contacts with prominent oncologists in the region. I have achieved Board Certification in Medical Affairs (BCMAS) as evidence of my dedication to the field. I am eager to engage in a conversation on this role with you.

Sincerely,
Suzanne Soliman

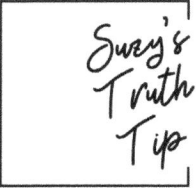

When you're applying for MSL jobs, it's important to tailor your CV and cover letter to the specific role. Highlight the skills and experience that are most relevant to the job, and use keywords that are relevant to the industry.

Request for a Letter of Reference

When reaching out to an individual, such as a past professor, for a letter of reference or recommendation, it is important to do so with professionalism and etiquette. You can follow the template below when writing your own request.

Esteemed Dr./Professor [Individual's Last Name],

Greetings, I trust this email reaches you in good health. I am [Your Name], and I was a student enrolled in your [Name of Course] course during the [Semester/Year]. [I was a resident in your residency program.] I am writing to formally solicit a letter of recommendation from you to endorse my candidacy for [Name of program/scholarship/opportunity/position].

As you may remember, I enthusiastically engaged in class debates and consistently received high grades. I found your lectures on [specific topic] to be especially enlightening, and I successfully incorporated those insights into my [project/presentation/ assignment]. Your mentorship and motivation not only facilitated my outstanding performance in your course but also nurtured my enthusiasm for [subject of interest].

I am presently seeking admission to the [program/scholarship/ opportunity/position] due to its congruence with my objectives and aspirations. I am confident that the skills and knowledge I acquired in your class, particularly [specify relevant abilities or knowledge pertaining to the opportunity], will be crucial for my achievement in this undertaking.

I acknowledge that composing a letter of reference necessitates a significant amount of work and exertion, and I genuinely value your willingness to help me. For your convenience, I have sent my CV and a transcript for your reference. I am willing to furnish any supplementary information that you may require. The reference letter must be submitted by [date].

Thank you for dedicating your time and thoughtful consideration. I anticipate receiving a prompt response from you.

Yours faithfully,

[Your Name]
[Contact Details]

The following is not required or mandatory, but you may cite particular occurrences in which you left a strong impression on the professor, such as surpassing expectations in an assignment or making substantial contributions to class discussions. If you had any extracurricular engagement with the lecturer, briefly discuss that contact and explain how it further strengthened your passion for the subject. Ensure to meticulously revise your letter before sending it.

The Job Search Process

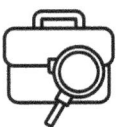

When you start exploring the job market, that is when you truly step into the realm of all the MSL positions that are open to you. Yet, finding a role that is a good fit for you requires a thoughtful approach. Here, I'll walk you through the process, from researching the MSL roles and identifying companies that align with your aspirations to building meaningful connections within the industry. Let's start your MSL job hunt with renewed confidence and clarity!

The Role of Keywords in MSL Job Searches

A keyword is a word or phrase that is used to describe a specific job or skill. Keywords are important in a job search because they can help you find jobs that are relevant to your skills and experience. When you search for jobs online, you can use keywords to narrow down your search results. For example, if you are looking for a job in the medical field, you could use keywords like "medical," "healthcare," and "doctor."

Employers also use keywords to find qualified candidates. When an employer posts a job opening, they will often include a list of keywords in the job description. These keywords are used by Applicant Tracking Systems (ATS) to scan resumes and identify candidates who match the skills and experience that the employer is looking for.

List of Essential Keywords

First, let's start with keywords for MSLs. Here are some keywords that you should have in your resume for a Medical Science Liaison.:

- Medical Science Liaison
- MSL
- Clinical research
- Pharmaceutical industry
- Drug development
- Healthcare
- Medical Education
- Scientific communication
- Relationship management
- Teamwork
- Problem-solving
- Data analysis
- Presentation skills

- Writing skills
- Influencing skills

Some Useful Resources

Staying on top of the latest news in the pharma/biotech industries can boost your confidence and readiness for a job interview; you can gain insights into how companies are performing and discover new companies and opportunities. Plus, being well-informed will allow you to craft insightful responses during interviews. Additionally, take advantage of the resources provided below.

One of my top recommendations for those interested in medical affairs and careers in this field is the Association of Clinical Medical Affairs (ACMA). Their resources are invaluable for anyone looking to excel in this area.

Take advantage of the news resources I have compiled below:

- ACMA: https://medicalaffairsspecialist.org/blog
- Medical Science Liaisons: https://medicalscienceliaison.org
- Pharmaceutical Executive: https://www.pharmexec.com
- PharmaVoice: https://www.pharmavoice.com
- Fierce Pharma: https://www.fiercepharma.com
- BioSpace: https://www.biospace.com
- BioPharma Dive: https://www.biopharmadive.com
- STAT News: https://www.statnews.com
- Endpoints News: https://endpts.com

- Wall Street Journal Health Industry Blog: https://www.wsj.com/news/business/health-industry
- Bloomberg Pharmaceutical Industry Blog: https://www.bloomberg.com/markets/sectors/health-care
- Pharmacy Times: https://www.pharmacytimes.com

You can also look up various company and investor websites as well. Here are some examples:

- https://ir.marinuspharma.com/investors/default.aspx
- https://investors.pfizer.com/Investors/Overview
- https://news.us.sumitomo-pharma.com
- https://investor.ironwoodpharma.com/home/default.aspx
- https://www.merck.com/investor-relations

The following databases will provide you with comprehensive information on clinical trials, drug development, and regulatory updates:

- The Pink Sheet: https://pink.citeline.com
- Clinicaltrials.gov: https://clinicaltrials.gov
- National Institute of Health: https://www.nih.gov
- U.S. Food and Drug Administration: https://www.fda.gov

You can also follow the following social media pages:

- *Suzanne Soliman*: Award-winning board-certified pharmacist, professor, global speaker, co-editor of *A Pharmacist Parent's Guide to Work-Life Balance,* author of *The Ultimate Guide to Becoming a Medical Science Liaison (MSL)*

- TikTok Channel:
  https://www.tiktok.com/@drsuzannesoliman

- Instagram Channel:
  https://www.instagram.com/drsuzannesoliman

- YouTube Channel:
  https://www.youtube.com/@drsuzannesoliman

- *William Soliman:* Founder/CEO of the ACMA

  - TikTok Channel:
    https://www.tiktok.com/@willsoliman

  - YouTube Channel:
    https://www.youtube.com/@willsoliman

Identifying Target Companies

Once you have a good understanding of the MSL role, you'll need to identify your target companies—those developing products you are interested in or have a strong reputation for MSL training and development.

There are several ways to identify target companies. You can look at the websites of pharmaceutical companies, read industry publications, and attend industry events. You can also use online job boards such as LinkedIn to search for MSL positions.

To identify target firms for job prospects, it is important to have a clear knowledge of your career objectives and actively search for organizations that provide positions in line with your talents and interests. Below is a review of suggestions for the pharmaceutical industry and other sectors.

Conventional pharmaceuticals:

Wholesale and distribution companies in the healthcare industry include McKesson, Cardinal Health, and AmerisourceBergen. These companies encompass positions in the management of medicine supply chains, procurement, and quality assurance.

Consider exploring opportunities in pharmaceutical corporations and biotech firms within the field of Research and Development. These roles may involve tasks such as drug discovery, conducting clinical studies, and managing regulatory affairs. Seek managerial roles in pharmacy operations, quality assurance, or medication information across diverse healthcare environments. Specialty Pharmacy: Seek positions in illness management, patient education, and medication adherence programs offered by specialty pharmacies.

Big Pharma refers to large, established pharmaceutical companies that often have extensive resources and capabilities. Big Pharma companies often operate on a broad scale, developing drugs for various therapeutic areas and diseases. They are multinational corporations with substantial financial resources, extensive organizational structure, and a broad portfolio of marketed drugs. Big Pharma companies tend to have a more stable revenue stream from existing drugs. The profitability is often driven by their blockbuster drugs, which have a large market potential.

Pharmaceutical companies that go beyond the ordinary:

- **Medical equipment companies:** Medtronic, Abbott Laboratories, Siemens Healthineers. Explore opportunities in clinical research, product development, regulatory affairs, or sales that include supporting medical devices used in patient care.

- **Biotechnology companies:** Biotechnology refers to the field that combines biology and technology to develop drugs, therapies, and diagnostic tools. They mainly focus on areas such as genomics, proteomics, targeted drug delivery, immunotherapy, or gene therapy. Biotech companies are generally more specialized and focus on specific areas of research. They often leverage cutting-edge scientific techniques and technologies to develop novel therapies or diagnostic tools. The success of a biotech company largely depends on the approval and commercial success of its pipeline products. Some prominent biotech companies are Amgen, Gilead Sciences, and Celgene. Discover prospects in the fields of clinical research, drug development, regulatory affairs, or the commercialization of innovative products and therapies.

- **Consulting Firms:** These include companies specializing in providing advice and guidance in the healthcare industry, specifically in areas such as pharmaceutical benefit management. Seek positions focused on enhancing efficiency in pharmacy operations, implementing medication adherence programs, or conducting healthcare policy analysis.

- **Government Agencies:** The Food and Drug Administration (FDA) and the Centers for Medicare & Medicaid Services (CMS). Seek positions in the field of drug regulation, policy formulation, or public health initiatives pertaining to pharmaceuticals.

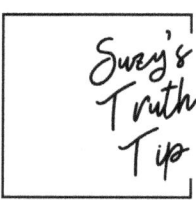

Remember, before you even start applying for jobs, make sure to thoroughly research what the role of an MSL entails and understand the pharmaceutical industry as a whole! I can't emphasize this enough. Understanding these aspects will help you tailor your CV and cover letter to align perfectly with the job and industry requirements.

Key Strategies for an Effective Job Search

To effectively navigate the job search process in the industry, it's essential to employ a strategic approach—maintain flexibility in your choices, engage in proactive networking, and adapt your job search according to your developing professional objectives and current market conditions.

Networking and Research

- **Participate and communicate:** Engage across various industries, attend conferences, and leverage organizations like the American Pharmacists Association (APhA) or the American Medical Association (AMA) to establish connections.

- **Employment Listings and Company Websites:** Utilize available resources such as LinkedIn, APhA's career center, and specific company job boards to identify relevant opportunities.

- **Study Organizational Culture:** Gain insights into the work environment and values through reviews, corporate websites, and interactions with current employees.

- **Utilize relevant professional groups in social media:** Utilize various professional groups on LinkedIn or Facebook as a means to establish connections with individuals in your industry. Engage in pertinent communities, actively contribute to conversations, and initiate contact with persons who pique your interest. By utilizing this, you might get knowledge about concealed prospects and establish a remarkable impact on prospective employers.

Customizing Application Materials

- **Optimize your CV and cover letter:** Devote sufficient time to thoroughly examine the job description and customize your CV and cover letter to precisely match the specified requirements. Ensure consistency in the information provided, including your name, email address, phone number, and LinkedIn profile URL. Don't forget to incorporate relevant keywords in your documents to increase the visibility of your application.

- **Optimize online profile in company portals/job boards:** Optimize your online presence by developing a robust profile that effectively highlights your competencies, expertise, and notable accomplishments. Utilize pertinent keywords to enhance the discoverability of your profile by recruiters.

Navigating Online Job Boards

A job board is where companies advertise their job openings. While this is an invaluable tool for hiring managers and recruiters, it is also vital for prospective job seekers. You can streamline your job search process by easily identifying positions that align with your skills and preferences.

- **Focus your search:** Online job boards can be a valuable resource in your job hunt, but it is crucial to use them efficiently. Focus your search using sophisticated search filters to refine your choices based on region, job type, industry, pay, range, and/or other parameters.

- **Consider the geographical location and salary offered:** Avoid indiscriminately applying to every job you encounter. Focus on harmonizing professional ambitions with location preferences and target wage range. For instance, if you are aware that you reside in Chicago and have no intention of relocating from Chicago, it would be unnecessary to conduct employment searches throughout the entire United States. There is no purpose or reason. By selectively extracting and employing the necessary information, you will optimize your time and guarantee that you encounter the pertinent opportunities. If you specifically desire remote work, refrain from searching for office jobs.

- **Create job alerts:** Ensure your competitive advantage by configuring email notifications for newly available positions that align with your specific requirements. By doing this, you will ensure that you do not overlook any prospective possibilities.

The titles for positions within the MSL role can differ from one company to another. These titles may include:[18]

- Clinical Science Liaison
- Clinical Science Manager
- Clinical Trial Liaison
- Country Medical Director*
- Field Medical Director
- Health Science Associate

- Managed Care Liaison
- Medical Advisor
- Medical Affairs Liaison
- Medical Development Manager
- Medical Education Research Liaison
- Medical Information Scientist
- Medical Liaison
- Medical Liaison Director
- Medical Manager*
- Medical Rep*
- Medical Science Manager
- MSL Trainer
- National Medical Scientist
- Patient Care Liaisons
- Professional Education Liaison
- Regional Associate Director
- Regional Clinical Science Liaison
- Regional Medical Advisor
- Regional Medical Associate
- Regional Medical Director
- Regional Medical Liaison
- Regional Scientific Manager
- Scientific Affairs Liaison

*International titles may vary; medical reps may often hold advanced degrees.

Exhibiting Professionalism

Consistently demonstrate a professional demeanor in all your interactions, whether they occur online or offline. This will create a favorable impression on prospective employers and colleagues. It is important to keep in mind that properly utilizing an online job board requires continuous effort.

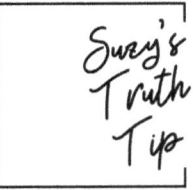

The job search process can be long and challenging, but it's important to be persistent. Keep applying for jobs, even if you don't get the first few that you apply for. Eventually, you'll find the right role for you.

Efficient Networking at Industry Events

Attending industry events, conferences, and networking events can be valuable for MSL professionals at any stage of their careers. While it can be a source of anxiety for many to find the right people to talk to and start a conversation, communication and networking skills are crucial to help your personal and professional development. It's essential to look for events relevant to your field and beneficial to your future endeavors.

Prior to the event:

- **Establish your objectives:** Determine what you want to achieve from the event. Are you searching for employment, establishing professional relationships, or acquiring knowledge about current developments in the field? Having a clear understanding of your objectives will help you focus your efforts.

- **Research Attendees and Speakers:** Who is presenting at the event? Which individuals are attending? What sessions or workshops are available? Identify key individuals you would like to connect with or learn from. Research their background, current projects, and any recent publications or achievements. This will help you identify potential connections and opportunities more effectively.

- **Engage on Social Media:** Join relevant groups or discussions on platforms like LinkedIn or X related to the event. Engaging with other attendees beforehand can help break the ice and establish initial connections.

- **Prepare your elevator pitch:** When initiating conversation, it's important to approach with confidence and, at the same time, with kindness. Create and rehearse a compelling introduction about yourself, highlighting your expertise, experience, and what you seek from the event. Brainstorm some conversation starters and topics that tie to the theme of the event.

- **Ensure you carry business cards:** Make sure you have sufficient business cards to exchange with fellow attendees.

The cards should feature your contact details and website/ LinkedIn profile.

- **Adhere to an appropriate dress code:** To make a solid first impression, it's important to choose attire that suits the event.

Throughout the event:

- **Take initiative:** Don't be afraid to initiate conversations with other attendees. Approach them with a smile and introduce yourself with your prepared elevator pitch. Engage with the attendees during appropriate seminars, poster presentations, or networking breaks.

- **Engage in active listening:** Focus your attention on the words and ideas expressed by others and seek to establish shared interests or topics for discussion. Ask insightful questions and show genuine interest in their work or experiences.

- **Provide added value:** Avoid solely focusing on self-promotion. Instead, share your expertise, specialized knowledge, and valuable perspectives. Offer assistance or advice when suitable. This approach not only enhances your credibility but also enriches interactions by fostering meaningful exchanges.

- **Exchange contact information:** After a meaningful conversation, exchange business cards or connect on LinkedIn to stay in touch. Consider jotting down relevant notes on the back of received business cards to remember key points about the individual.

- **Engage with a wide range of individuals:** Avoid exclusively targeting high-ranking executives. Anyone has the potential to become a valued connection.

- **Participate in social gatherings:** Numerous events feature receptions or dinners. They provide informal environments for socializing with people in a laid-back atmosphere. If you tend to be an introverted person, this can be daunting yet necessary. Set a time limit and allow oneself grace to bow out after an hour or two. Alternatively, set a goal to make one meaningful connection and allow permission to exit once that goal is met!

- **Show consideration for others' time:** Ensure that your introductions and chats are brief and to the point, particularly when attending crowded events.

After the event:

- **Follow Up Promptly:** To maintain contact and further develop your initial connections, send personalized follow-up emails or LinkedIn messages within a few days of the event. Express your appreciation for the conversation and reiterate any points discussed.

- **Maintain Relationships:** Keep in touch with your new contacts periodically. Share relevant articles, updates, or industry insights to add value to your relationship.

- **Join professional organizations:** Become a member of industry groups or societies to expand your professional network and open doors to new possibilities.

- **Reflect on Insights:** Take some time to reflect on the insights gained and lessons learned from the event. Consider how you can apply this knowledge to your work or career goals.

Keep in mind that networking involves establishing connections and fostering relationships rather than simply collecting business cards. Direct your attention towards establishing authentic relationships, and you will have a higher probability of experiencing advantageous outcomes in the future.

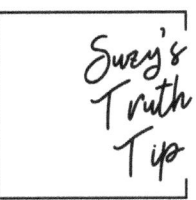

Networking with current and former MSLs is a great way to learn more about the role and to get your foot in the door. Attend industry events, connect with MSLs on LinkedIn, and reach out to people in your network who may know someone who is an MSL.

Small Versus Large Companies: What's Better for First-Time MSLs?

Both small and large companies offer unique opportunities and challenges for first-time Medical Science Liaisons (MSLs).[19] Choosing between them depends on various factors, including individual preferences, career goals, and personal circumstances. There are always exceptions to any rule; however, larger companies often have more resources to invest in training new MSLs, to provide in-depth disease state training, or business-oriented job specifics. Conversely, a small company may not have such capacity. They may, therefore, often lean towards hiring someone with job experience and/or who is considered a leader or expert in the disease state. It is just less likely for a new company to hire a person without MSL experience. A contract MSL position is another option worth considering, as it could provide you with valuable experience you can leverage for a full-time opportunity in the future.

Here's a breakdown of the advantages and considerations for each:

	Small Companies/ Start-ups	Large Companies/ Corporations
Sizes and Financial Earnings:	Generally characterized by having less than 500 employees and yearly sales below $1 billion. Frequently centered on specialized markets or cultivating distinct, pioneering therapies.	Typically employ tens of thousands of individuals and generate yearly revenue in the billions. Frequently possess varied portfolios encompassing numerous therapeutic areas and well-established brands.
Organizational Structure and Decision-making:	Typically have a flatter hierarchy, allowing for quicker decision-making and increased flexibility. Employees assume various roles and possess greater responsibility for projects.	Often have departments that operate independently, which can lead to slower decision-making and a reliance on established systems. Roles are highly specialized, resulting in reduced individual impact for employees.

	Small Companies/ Start-ups	Large Companies/ Corporations
Research and Development (R&D):	Small enterprises in this context typically prioritize early-stage development and the practice of licensing their discoveries to larger corporations. Can collaborate with academic institutions or contract research organizations.	Large companies possess comprehensive in-house R&D capacities that span all aspects of the drug development process, ranging from initial discovery to final product launch. May possess greater financial resources and more extensive capabilities for conducting clinical trials.
Marketing and Sales:	Utilize focused marketing strategies to reach certain Healthcare Professionals (HCPs) and Key Opinion Leaders (KOLs). Direct sales teams often consist of a smaller number of individuals and are typically limited to specific geographic regions.	Large companies typically implement global marketing campaigns with larger sales teams operating on a global scale.

	Small Companies/ Start-ups	**Large Companies/ Corporations**
Advantages:	1. May provide valuable hands-on experience in various aspects of medical affairs beyond typical MSL duties, contributing to diverse skills. 2. Due to the entrepreneurial environment, employees have a more significant impact by having direct access to key decision-makers and the opportunity to shape the medical strategy of the company.	1. Many large pharmaceutical companies offer comprehensive training programs for MSLs. 2. Large companies typically have well-established resources and support systems for MSLs, i.e., medical information databases and internal experts. 3. Provides access to a broader network.

Board Certification

As the landscape of medical affairs continues to evolve, the need for standardized training has become increasingly apparent. In a competitive field where standing out is essential, board certifications and fellowships offer a tangible way to enhance credibility, demonstrate expertise, and gain a competitive advantage. But how do you choose which is the right one for you? Let's find out!

BCMAS Certification

Since 2015, the number of MSLs has increased significantly and with that explosion there has been a similar increase in the number of people who want to become MSLs. That has created fierce competition among candidates wanting to enter the MSL profession. Additionally, the skill set needed to be a successful MSL nowadays has changed as well with a greater emphasis on having a broad set of skills and knowledge across the medical affairs, medical information, and MSL landscape. To this end, in 2015, there was the development of the first ever Board Certification for MSLs. Currently, the official Board Certification program for MSLs is the Board Certified Medical Affairs Specialist (BCMAS) program which is governed by the ACMA.

The BCMAS certification is a valuable credential because it is recognized by employers in the pharmaceutical industry.[20] Offered by ACMA, the BCMAS program is also globally recognized in the healthcare industry and accredited by International Accreditors for Continuing Education and Training (IACET). To be eligible for a BCMAS designation, individuals must hold a terminal degree (MD, PhD, DO, DNP or PharmD). This comprehensive program includes 20 modules of content that cover:

- All stages of product development
- The roles/responsibilities of MSLs
- Clinical research
- Regulatory compliance
- Medical Affairs
- Publication practices
- Abstract/medical writing
- Medical Education
- Data analysis
- Rules on interactions with healthcare providers and KOLs
- The payer landscape
- Business strategies
- Soft skills like teamwork, communication, critical thinking, and problem-solving

The program requires MSLs to complete a series of self-assessments, case studies, and exams. This process helps MSLs identify their strengths and weaknesses and develop strategies for improving their performance.

Many employers view the BCMAS certification as a sign of an MSL's commitment to their professional development, and they may be more likely to hire an MSL who has the certification. In an ACMA survey, 87% of KOLs responded that MSLs who held BCMAS were perceived as being more credible, trustworthy, and competent than their non-certified counterparts. [21] The majority of KOLs agreed that it demonstrates the company's commitment to excellence in patient quality and care. According to a survey by the Medical Science Liaison Society, 75% of MSLs who are certified with BCMAS believe that the certification has helped them advance their careers. The survey also found that 80% of employers believe that the BCMAS certification is a valuable credential for MSLs.

A great way to increase your relevance in the industry is to gain knowledge and become certified in the field. Obtaining a Board Certified Medical Affairs Specialist (BCMAS) certification to add to your CV significantly enhances your competitive edge among other candidates. It shows your commitment to furthering your expertise in medical affairs and the MSL role. In fact, 90% of physician thought leaders prefer a BCMAS candidate when looking to fill open roles.[20]

Here's how a BCMAS certification can boost your career:[22]

- **A BCMAS certification is a testament to your expertise:** Accuracy in medical information holds the utmost importance in sectors like pharmaceuticals. Board certification serves as a rigorous standard that confirms your expertise, professional competence, and extensive knowledge in medical science, pharmacology, and relevant therapy areas.

- **It is an assurance of your ethical commitment:** The pharmaceutical industry has its fair share of challenges that invite scrutiny, whether due to questionable promotional tactics or unintentional misinformation. Board certification is like a badge of honor that showcases your commitment to upholding a strict code of ethics, promoting transparency, ensuring accountability, and placing patient well-being above any commercial interests.

- **Board certification serves as a cornerstone of trust:** Having a board certification empowers Medical Science Liaisons and Medical Affairs Professionals by bolstering trust and credibility in collaborative efforts and facilitating more informed treatment decisions.

- **A board certification places you on par with other certified healthcare specialists:** This recognition not only validates your expertise but also integrates you into a committed and proficient professional network, thus enhancing your career prospects.

Globally, numerous organizations provide board certification for MSL and Medical Affairs professionals, underscoring the pharmaceutical industry's dedication to excellence. Among these, BCMAS stands out as a comprehensive option. For those aspiring to a career as an MSL, BCMAS certification serves as a valuable credential, setting candidates apart from their peers and propelling career advancement.

The Medical Affairs Competency Certificate

If you are currently in a doctorate-level program and interested in becoming an MSL but are not yet eligible for BCMAS, there is another route for you. The Medical Affairs Competency Certificate (MACC) is the go-to program that will get you ahead in the pharmaceutical industry. This accredited program allows students to master information about Medical Science Liaisons and Field-Based Medical Teams. Comprising seven comprehensive modules, the program is completely online and self-paced![23]

The modules cover:

- Pharmaceutical Industry Overview
- Rules Governing Interactions with Healthcare Providers
- Regulatory Affairs
- Overview of Compliance
- Drug Development and Lifecycle Management
- Medical Science Liaisons & Field-Based Medical Teams
- Diversity in Clinical Trials

MSL Post-Doctoral Fellowships

An industry pathway to break out into this role is through a post-doctoral fellowship. Many pharmaceutical companies have partnered with universities, such as Rutgers University and Northeastern University, to provide the opportunity for graduates from MD, DO, and PharmD programs to work in the industry.

Many companies like Novo Nordisk and Eli Lilly have also created such programs but without any university affiliation.[23] In 2020-2021, the Industry Pharmacists Organization (IPhO) conducted an analysis revealing that approximately 83 companies within their fellowship cohort supported post-doctoral fellowships.[24] These fellowships were either independently managed or affiliated with universities.

Fellowship programs are designed to provide participants with opportunities to develop core competencies in field-based scientific exchange of medical information. The programs also allow fellows to learn about the pharmaceutical industry through cross-functional work across various departments, i.e., Medical Affairs, Marketing, Regulatory Affairs, Legal, Safety, and Health Outcomes Research.

Joining cross-disciplinary teams helps new graduates boost their communication skills. Meanwhile, taking on a post-doctoral fellowship opens doors to unique career opportunities where you can polish essential soft skills needed to stand out in a competitive job market.

While a post-doctoral fellowship is not necessary to work in this field, it provides strong mentorship and opportunities if you're looking to gain experience in the industrial setting. Throughout the structured one to two-year post-doctoral fellowship program, graduates can work closely with preceptors and mentors to develop specific skills in the functional area. Graduates will solidify their skills for a post-fellowship position as a medical affairs specialist.

Suzy's Truth Tip

Get the right experience! While there is no one-size-fits-all educational or professional background for an MSL, most employers look for candidates with a Ph.D. or MD in a relevant field, as well as experience in clinical research or medical communications. If you don't have the right experience, you can still get your foot in the door by getting involved in extracurricular activities or volunteering your time to work with healthcare professionals.

Acing Your Interview: Before, During, and After

Your job search strategy paid off, and your preparation met the opportunity: the interview! Interviewing for MSL positions is a multi-step process that may span several weeks. It may seem nerve-wracking, but proceeding strategically and confidently can greatly increase your chances of success. In this chapter, I will break down each stage of the interview process so that you are well-equipped to leave a strong impression on hiring managers!

The MSL Hiring Process

When it comes to landing that MSL job, acing the job interview is crucial. Familiarizing yourself with common interview setups can greatly smooth out the process. Typically, the hiring process can extend over a significant period, often lasting more than a month.

Though each company might have its own way of conducting interviews, most MSL interviews follow a typical format. Offering an important opportunity for you to shine and demonstrate why you're the best candidate, the hiring process generally unfolds in three stages:

1. **Phone Screening:** You'll speak with a member of the HR or talent acquisition team. This is an opportunity for them to get to know you better and determine whether you're a suitable match for the position.

2. **Face-to-Face Interview:** The next interview could take place either face-to-face or virtually, allowing you to connect with the hiring manager. This is your opportunity to delve deeper into your skills, expertise, and experiences.

3. **Clinical Paper Presentation:** Finally, you may be asked to prepare and present a clinical paper. This opportunity allows you to showcase your expertise in the field and demonstrate your skill in communicating complex clinical data effectively.

Preparing for the Interview

Well done! You have successfully secured a phone interview for a Medical Science Liaison (MSL) role. There is a sense of anticipation accompanied by a slight feeling of hesitation. Don't be afraid; this chapter will function as a guide, directing you through the phone screening and interview phases as you progress toward being a reliable scientific intermediary.

Preparation in advance is the secret to a successful interview. Maximize your interview by gaining as much knowledge as possible about the organization beforehand. Preparation is crucial because it makes you appear comprehensive, professional, and enthusiastic about the position. It also enables you to ask better questions, increasing your chances of obtaining the necessary information to evaluate the position.

1. **Know the Interview Format:** Understand whether the interview will be in person or virtual. Request crucial details such as duration, date, time, and location. Most companies will give you an itinerary prior to your interview, while some will provide it upon your arrival.

2. **Research the Company Thoroughly:** Beyond superficial browsing, delve deeply into the company's background. Explore their website. Usually, the company will have press releases and investor webcasts/webinars posted on their site (click the "investors" tab), which are usually for equity research analysts, investors, etc. Take note of their leadership priorities, how they pronounce key drug names (yes, I'm serious), and common questions addressed during these sessions. Additionally, gather information on the company's location, facility type, organizational structure, reputation, strategic plans, and fiscal updates. Stay updated on any expansions, stock values, or plans to go public. Financial news and investment journals are the best sources for this.

3. **Research the Pipeline and Key Opinion Leaders (KOLs):** Examine the company's pipeline and publications associated with the pipeline product. Identify authors of relevant research papers, as they will most likely be the KOLs (known as External Experts or Key Thought Leaders as well). Look them up online, often on platforms like YouTube, or look for guidelines they've authored for that specific therapeutic field.

Study the guidelines to understand the disease state and the new product. Strategically mention what you learned during your interview to impress the interviewers. Also, familiarize yourself with recent FDA approvals and press releases related to the company.

4. **Understand the Interviewer(s):** Research the background and expertise of your interviewers, tailoring your responses to align with their interests and team dynamics. Leverage your network to gather insights from current or past employees of the organization. Try to call your interviewers by their last name and avoid using their first names; for example, Dr. Jane Warner would be Dr. Warner rather than Jane.

5. **Practice "Tell me about yourself":** This would be your elevator pitch, and it would be your first impression. You have only seven seconds to make that first impression. Craft the "Tell me about yourself" question by highlighting your strengths and aligning them with the role's requirements. Keep it concise, focusing on recent professional accomplishments. This should be a quick one to two-minute response, not something that takes eight minutes or refers to things very far in your past, like being the captain of your high school soccer team. Consider sharing your short-term and long-term goals. Short-term goals are intended to be achieved within 1-2 years while long-term goals are typically 3 years or more ahead of the time.

6. **Practice Makes Perfect:** Conduct mock interviews with friends, colleagues, or career coaches to refine your responses and boost your confidence.

7. **Prepare Questions:** Demonstrate your genuine interest by having thoughtful questions about the team, company culture, and specific challenges they face.

8. **Pay Attention to Logistics:** If it's an in-person interview, plan your travel meticulously and dress professionally. Be punctual, arriving at least 10-15 minutes early. For virtual interviews, ensure a stable internet connection and a quiet, well-lit environment.

9. **Demonstrate Professionalism:** Maintain professionalism throughout the interview process, from your initial handshake (if in person) to your communication style. Address interviewers respectfully, using appropriate titles.

Imagine you've impressed the interviewer in your first screening! Now, it's time to meet the MSL hiring manager and team. Whether it's an in-person or virtual setting, this chapter will equip you with the tools to showcase your MSL brilliance and shine during the interview.

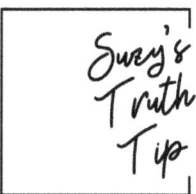

Here are tips on addressing questions and concerns that may arise during the interview:

1. *Why are you leaving your current job?*
   Do not badmouth your current employer. Instead, focus on what this job offers that your old job did not!

2. *Tell us about the gaps in your resume.*
   A polite way to answer this is to share how much time you spent focusing on a personal project. They do not need to know the details. Try to focus on things that are beneficial for this new role, such as the courses you took or the certifications you have received!

3. *Why do you want the job?*
   We all want to be paid. Hiring managers do not want to hear that you want it because you get to work from home and get a good salary. Instead, offer a genuine interest in the position or company.

4. *What is your current salary?*
   Do not let them know because this could be an issue, and it is illegal in certain states to ask this. It could be detrimental when you are negotiating, and what you are currently paid should be based on the current rate and market rate based on your skills.

The Phone Screening

The phone screening process is usually implemented by large or global pharmaceutical companies with well-established recruitment protocols. It is a preliminary phase, typically facilitated by a Human Resources or Talent Acquisition representative, who engages in a brief, informal conversation with the candidate lasting around 10 to 15 minutes. This presents a chance to create a powerful initial impact by demonstrating your enthusiasm and suitability for the position. The recruiter or HR representative will evaluate the following:

1. *Minimum qualifications:* Are you able to fulfill the essential requirements outlined in the job description? Are you eligible to work based on citizenship or visa?

2. *Communication skills:* Are you able to express your opinions with clarity and brevity? Do you possess a sincere passion for the MSL role and the company's mission?

During the Phone Screen:

To ensure a seamless interview, prepare yourself by following these steps:

- *Professionalism and Politeness:* Begin the phone screen with a warm greeting, ensuring you convey professionalism and politeness throughout the conversation. Articulate your responses clearly and confidently.

- *Active Listening and Concise Responses:* Focus closely on each question asked, providing concise and relevant answers. Do not go off-topic.

- *Highlight Relevant Skills and Experiences:* Tailor your responses to highlight the skills and experiences that directly align with the requirements of the MSL position. Showcase your ability to excel in the role.

- *Demonstrate Enthusiasm:* Express genuine excitement for the opportunity to work as a Medical Science Liaison. Share your passion for the field and convey how it aligns with your career aspirations.

- *Ask Thoughtful Questions:* Demonstrate your interest in the organization and the role by posing insightful questions. This not only showcases your initiative but also displays your understanding of the company culture and expectations.

- *Follow-Up With Gratitude:* After the phone screen, send a follow-up email to thank the interviewer for their time and consideration. Reiterate your enthusiasm for the role and express your continued interest in moving forward in the hiring process.

The Interview

The interview is usually conducted by either the hiring manager or a member of the MSL team, typically the MSL Manager or Medical Manager. This could be in-person or virtual, lasts about an hour, and focuses on your background, expertise, and personality, delving into your skills through behavioral questions. During the interview, they'll look into a few key areas to better understand your expertise and abilities in the therapeutic field. Secondly, they'll assess how effectively you can communicate complex medical knowledge, which is crucial for effective communication in this field.

Getting Ready for the Interview:

- *Expand your understanding of the therapeutic field* by focusing on recent advancements, relevant clinical trials, key medications, and important clinical protocols/guidelines.

- *Be prepared to address technical inquiries* by anticipating questions about disease mechanisms, mode of action for medications, and clinical trial findings.

- *Compile and create case studies* to skillfully convey complex medical concepts clearly and concisely to individuals without scientific backgrounds.

- *Conduct a thorough research of the interview panel* to gain insights into their backgrounds and areas of expertise.

- *Prepare answers for key questions* such as why you're drawn to the MSL position, your knowledge of the company, your grasp of the MSL role, your potential contributions, your methods for staying updated on clinical research, the toughest part of your current job, and what sets you apart from other applicants.

During the Phone Interview:

- *Showcase your scientific proficiency:* Provide meticulous and precise answers to technical questions, showcasing your scientific expertise and proficiency in the field.

- *Utilize storytelling and analogies:* Explain complex concepts in a clear and relatable manner, rendering them accessible and comprehensible.

- *Highlight your communication skills:* Actively listen, ask for further clarification if needed, and tailor your responses to suit your specific audience.

- *Showcase your interpersonal skills:* Share instances where you've excelled in working collaboratively, tackling intricate challenges, and using analytical reasoning to solve complex problems.

- *Ask insightful questions:* This showcases your inquisitiveness and readiness.

- *Send a follow-up email:* It is a great opportunity to express gratitude and appreciation while highlighting your qualifications politely and courteously.

Psychometric Test:

After the initial interview, certain companies might request a second round involving a psychometric test. These tests delve deeper into your strengths and weaknesses, examining aspects of your personality, your analytical or mathematical abilities, and how you solve complex problems.

Keep in mind that the phone screen and interview serve as crucial milestones in your journey toward becoming an MSL. To establish a lasting impression, it is important to demonstrate your unique value proposition by being well-prepared, competent, and passionate. Therefore, inhale deeply, have faith in your expertise, and overcome these challenges related to the screening with assurance!

Suzy's
Truth
Tip

The number one interview mistake I have seen others make is that they do not know enough about the company. There are many ways to do research! Scour their company website, find their social media pages to see what the company posts about, and read any articles about the company! You can also look at the LinkedIn company page to find out who works there and see if you have any mutual connections. KNOW the company you are interviewing with.

Interview Etiquette

The majority of your interviews will be conducted via a virtual platform like Zoom, Teams, or WebEx. You may also have interviews over the phone and in person. For virtual and phone interviews, make sure you are interviewing in a quiet place without any distractions.

- *Dress professionally* during your interview. Conservative colors are best, such as dark blue, black, or gray. Women should wear low-heeled pumps and hair in a professional, neat style. Men should make sure they have clean dress shoes on. When it comes to online interviews, you don't have to go all out with a suit and tie just for your phone screen. Think about wearing a nice shirt paired with a tie, and maybe add a jacket, button-down, blouse, or sweater. While they might not see your pants, it's still a good idea to wear something dressy from the waist down, just in case. It's all about making a professional impression while staying comfortable during your interview.

- *Make sure there is ample light.* If there aren't any windows, turn on as many lights as you can so the interviewer(s) can see your face.

- *Virtual screen backgrounds* may seem okay, but many times, they are distracting. I recommend using the blur feature to just blur the background rather than using a virtual background. Make sure no one can see your bed, kitchen table, wallpaper, etc., especially if you are living in an unkempt place.

Well done! You have arrived at the ultimate challenge: the MSL interview presentation. Seize this opportunity to demonstrate your profound scientific knowledge, exceptional communication skills, and talent for captivating an audience. This chapter provides you with the necessary tools and tactics to give an impactful presentation that successfully secures your desired MSL job.

Interacting with the Recruiters

MSL recruiters are experts in finding and hiring suitable professionals for key positions in pharmaceutical, biotechnology, and medical device firms. To make the most of your interactions with MSL recruiters, it's crucial to be well-prepared and maintain a professional demeanor. Here are some helpful tips for effectively connecting with MSL recruiters:

- *Be ready:* Start by thoroughly researching the firm, the recruiter, and the exact MSL position you're interested in. Prepare to respond to inquiries regarding your abilities, professional background, and career aspirations.

- *Exhibit professionalism:* Ensure that you wear suitable attire for both phone conversations and face-to-face encounters. Exhibit politeness, courtesy, and enthusiasm consistently throughout the interaction.

- *Emphasize your proficiency and expertise:* Highlight your skills and expertise relevant to the MSL role. Use concrete examples and achievements to showcase your proficiency. Whenever possible, provide quantifiable data to support your accomplishments.

- *Ask insightful questions:* Showcase your enthusiasm and expertise by posing perceptive inquiries regarding the organization, the MSL team, and the specific position.

- *Express gratitude:* Thank the recruiter for their time following each interaction, and subsequently write a follow-up email after your interview to emphasize your continued interest in the position.

- *Exhibit candor and clarity:* Ensure that you are honest and accurate when describing your experience and qualifications. Avoid exaggerating your abilities or making unsupported assertions.

- *Exercise patience:* Be patient throughout the recruitment process, as it may be time-consuming. Stay organized by keeping track of your engagements with recruiters and organizations.

Avoid common pitfalls such as:

- Being ill-prepared or lacking knowledge about the firm or role.

- Exhibiting unprofessional behavior, such as inappropriate attire or language.

- Displaying negativity or criticism.

- Criticizing and speaking negatively about current and former employers/organizations.

- Asking about remuneration, benefits, or holidays prematurely.

- Having unrealistic expectations about the position. Show adaptability and a willingness to consider diverse prospects, even if they may not precisely align with your desired position.

- Ignoring emails or calls from recruiters.

- Responding with a harsh and negative demeanor to a hiring manager.

Focus on exuding confidence and enthusiasm for the field of research and healthcare. Network with other MSLs and professionals in the industry, stay informed about the latest developments in the pharmaceutical sector and utilize platforms like LinkedIn to showcase your expertise. Regardless of the outcome, remain courteous to anyone you interact with in the process, as the future is unpredictable, and you never know who you may meet again. By adhering to these guidelines and avoiding certain behaviors, you can create a favorable impression on Medical Science Liaison recruiters and enhance your prospects of securing your desired employment opportunity.

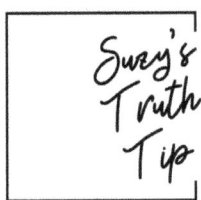

Communicate honestly and effectively with the recruiter. Be honest with the recruiter. They want you to get the job just as much as you want to get the job!

Interview Questions

You know by now that the Medical Science Liaison position plays a vital role in the pharmaceutical industry by providing education and support to healthcare professionals. As such, they are often subject to rigorous interview processes. I want you to prepare as much as possible for the interview by brainstorming answers to your questions and even practicing them in front of a mirror. You may even consider recording yourself to watch back your mannerisms and practice your questions again. Ask a friend or colleague to ask you some of the following questions from this chapter after you have rehearsed and ask for feedback. Good luck!

Potential Interview Questions

Here are some potential interview questions that you may be asked during a Medical Science Liaison job interview:

- *Tell me about yourself.* This is your chance to introduce yourself and highlight your relevant experience and skills.

Start with a brief overview of your professional background, focusing on key experiences in the pharmaceutical industry, your knowledge of clinical research, your achievements, and your ability to communicate effectively with healthcare professionals. Then, move to your current situation and why you're interested in the position or opportunity at hand. Finally, wrap up by expressing your enthusiasm for the role and how you believe your background aligns with the company's goals. Keep your answers focused on professional aspects and avoid personal details unless they directly relate to the job or company culture.

- *Tell me about your education, or walk me through your curriculum vitae.* This is a chance to discuss your history and how you got to where you are. Highlight any coursework or research experience directly related to the field of medical science or the therapeutic area of focus for the MSL role. Discuss any relevant internships, fellowships, or practical experiences that have prepared you for the responsibilities of an MSL.

- *Why are you interested in a career as an MSL?* This question is designed to assess your motivation for wanting to become an MSL. Be sure to talk about your interest in the pharmaceutical industry, your desire to educate healthcare professionals, and your passion for making a meaningful impact on patient care. Consider going more in-depth than the answer you would have prepared for the "Tell me about yourself" question.

- *What do you know about our company and our products?* This question is designed to assess how well you have researched the company, its competitors, customers, and innovations. Be sure to do your research before the interview so that you can answer this question intelligently.

- *What are your thoughts on the current state of the pharmaceutical industry?* This question is designed to assess your knowledge of the pharmaceutical industry and your ability to think critically about the challenges and opportunities facing the industry. Make sure you are up-to-date on various issues such as pricing, formularies, etc. Be mindful of stating any challenges in a positive light, and remember to refrain from saying anything negative or derogatory.

- *What is your experience with scientific communication?* This question is designed to assess your ability to communicate complex scientific information clearly and concisely. Be sure to talk about your experience with writing scientific papers, presenting at conferences, and communicating with healthcare professionals. This is important to demonstrate how you understand various therapeutic areas and also what is going on with the company.

- *How would you manage a difficult conversation with a healthcare professional?* The response to this question will enable the interviewer to assess your conflict resolution skills. Be sure to talk about your ability to remain calm and professional in difficult situations. Additionally, emphasize your strong communication skills, scientific expertise, and ability to build relationships, which are essential qualities for success in the MSL role. Consider having an example ready to share.

- *What are your thoughts on the role of MSLs in the pharmaceutical industry?* This question is designed to assess your understanding of the role of MSLs and your ability to think critically about the role.

- *Why are you a good fit for this role?* This question is important to show why you stand out compared to others.

- *Do you have experience working with KOLs?* This is to see if you are comfortable speaking with KOLs or if you have any relationships that can be used when you land the job. Who do you know? Who have you worked with in the past? How good are you at keeping connections and networking?

Ensure you can respond to queries on the following topics:

- Career Advancement
- Change Management
- Communication Abilities
- Conflict Resolution
- Using Creativity to Manage Criticism
- Decision-making Expertise
- Academic Experiences
- Time Management
- Problem-Solving

If you ever feel stuck, do not mention what you cannot do. Keep a positive attitude. Do not lie. Elaborate on an experience that you can use to relate to that skill and mention how you are a quick learner and have a thirst for knowledge.

These are just a few potential interview questions that you may be asked during a Medical Science Liaison job interview. Be sure to do your research, practice your answers, and dress professionally for your interview. Following these tips can increase your chances of acing your Medical Science Liaison interview.

In addition to the questions listed above, you may also be asked some technical questions about the pharmaceutical industry or the company's products. It is important to be prepared for these questions by doing your research and by reviewing the company's website and product information.

You may also be asked some behavioral questions. These questions are designed to assess your past behavior and how you would react in certain situations. Be sure to answer these questions honestly and provide specific examples from your experience.

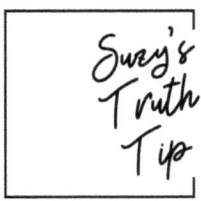

Practice your interviewing skills! Getting comfortable with interviewing is crucial. Once you start getting interviews, take time to practice your interviewing skills. This will help you feel more confident and prepared when you're in front of the interviewer.

Behavioral Questions

Most interviews rely heavily on behavioral questions to understand your approach to various situations. They aim to gauge your past behavior as an indicator of future performance. The most important way to respond to behavior-based questions is to be able to describe your situation in full and what you have learned from it.

For example, "Tell me about your strengths and weaknesses" is one of the most common behavioral interview questions. These questions are designed to elicit information about how you've handled past situations or how you might approach future ones. In the case of strengths and weaknesses, the interviewer is trying to measure your self-awareness, your ability to reflect on your skills and areas for improvement, and how you manage those weaknesses.

When responding to this type of question, it's important to be honest and provide examples or explanations to support your claims. For strengths, you might discuss specific skills or experiences that make you well-suited for the role. For weaknesses, be prepared to answer honestly with an area you have identified that you are actively working to improve or mitigate. Describe a positive change that has happened since you started working on it. This demonstrates self-awareness and a proactive approach to personal development. You do not have to discuss every single weakness you have.

Interviewers may also ask you about your leadership skills whether you are applying for a leadership position or not. Most of the time it is beneficial to use the term "we" did something vs "I" did something in order to show you have successfully worked with a team or on a team and that your team came out a success. It would be even more beneficial to describe the success of your team.

Other questions that a recruiter or hiring manager may ask are:

- Can you describe a time when you had to collaborate with a cross-functional team to achieve a goal?

- How do you handle difficult conversations or disagreements with KOLs?

- Can you give an example of a time when you had to manage multiple projects with competing deadlines?

- Give an example of a goal you've achieved and outline the steps you took to get there.

- How do you handle pressure? Give me an example.

- Describe a decision you made that was poorly received among colleagues. How did you implement it, and what was the result?

- Tell me about a time when you were able to inspire and motivate your team and/or colleagues.

Preparing for these questions using the STAR method (Situation, Task, Action, Result) and brainstorming three to four relevant scenarios beforehand can significantly boost your performance during the interview.

It is a fantastic approach you can use to tackle behavioral interview questions:

1. **Situation**: Describe the context or background of a specific situation or challenge you faced. Keep it brief, as you have limited time.

2. **Task**: Explain the particular task or goal you were aiming to accomplish.

3. **Action**: Outline the actions you took to address the task or overcome the challenge. Share a couple of key steps you found most impactful in achieving success. Even if your actions were taken as part of a team, avoid using "we" in your response and instead use "I" to highlight your particular contributions.

4. **Result**: Share the outcomes or results of your actions, including any lessons learned or achievements gained.

You should emphasize your strong work ethic and showcase your qualities like problem-solving, decision-making, leadership, enthusiasm, teamwork, and adaptability.

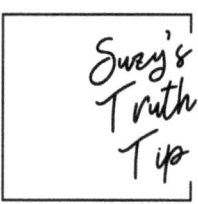

- *Prepare three to five stories that you can use for behavioral interview questions. Share the situation, your tasks, what you did, and how it helped the team or company.*

- *Prepare two to three questions to ask at the end of your interview.*

- *Make sure you remember to send a thank you email.*

What to Ask the Hiring Manager

As the interview comes to an end, anticipate the inevitable question: "Do you have any questions for us?" This moment is your opportunity to demonstrate your preparedness and understanding of both the company and the MSL role. Ask thoughtful inquiries that will allow you to learn information about the company that would not be readily accessible online.

The Medical Science Liaison job interview is a critical step in the hiring process. By being prepared and by answering the questions thoughtfully, you can increase your chances of landing the job.

Here are sample questions for the hiring manager:

- **About the role:**
  - What are the top three priorities of this role?
  - Could you describe the ideal candidate for this role?
  - What does a typical day look like for an MSL in this role?
  - What are the key challenges and opportunities of this role?
  - What is the reporting structure for this role?
  - What is the travel requirement for this role?
  - What kinds of assignments should I anticipate during the first 6 months of this position?
  - How soon will you be making a hiring decision?

- **About the company:**
  - What are the company's goals for the next year?
  - What are the company's strengths and weaknesses?
  - What do you like most about working for this company?
  - What is the company culture like?
  - What are the opportunities for advancement at this company?

- **About the MSL team:**
  - How many MSLs are on the team?
  - What is the team's philosophy on KOL engagement?
  - How does the team collaborate with other departments?
  - What is the team's culture like?
  - What is the projected growth of this team?
  - How closely do you work with other teams (medical, regulatory, marketing, etc.)?
  - What are the opportunities for professional development on the team?

These are just a few examples of questions a Medical Science Liaison candidate might ask a hiring manager. The specific questions you'll ask depend on your interests and experience. However, by asking thoughtful questions, you can show the hiring manager that you are serious about the role and that you have done your research. You can also use your questions to learn more about the company and the MSL team to see if this is a good fit for you.

What Not to Ask:

It's best to steer clear of certain topics to ensure the focus is on what truly matters. Here are a few things to keep in mind:

- *Money:* Do not bring up financial matters unless prompted. If asked, do not say, "I am currently making $98,000." Instead, inform that you are "actively interviewing for roles that pay between $140-180K" and if that is in line with the budget for this role. Wait to ask about the salary after you have been offered a position. Do not come out on the day of the interview and ask what your salary will be as you will NOT get you the job.

- *Vacations:* Similarly, avoid discussing vacations unless specifically asked. For example, do not let them know at this time that you need every Wednesday off because you play tennis.

- *Work-life balance:* Keep the conversation centered on your skills and contributions. Hiring managers aren't looking for people who are overly concerned with vacations and work-life balance. They prioritize individuals who are motivated and committed to the team's success.

- *Language use:* Avoid using casual expressions such as "like," "awesome," or "yeah." Maintaining a professional tone is key.

- *Etiquette:* Never smoke or chew gum during the interview – the same goes for sucking on a cough drop or hard candy. Refrain from checking your watch or cell phone. These actions can be distracting and detract from the conversation.

- *Avoid negativity:* Never criticize current or past employers, colleagues, or faculty members. Additionally, it's best to steer clear of discussions about controversial topics such as religion or politics.

The Interview Presentation

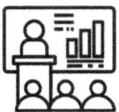

The interview presentation is the one last thing that is standing between you and your dream job! This is the platform where you can showcase your ability to present clinical data and critically appraise a clinical paper. But a presentation is not only about presenting the numbers; it is about how you present the numbers and how you tell the story behind the numbers. While your expertise and knowledge are unquestionable, perfecting the delivery is equally important. Worry not, as I am here to teach you how to architect and deliver an engaging presentation.

Strategies for a Dynamic and Compelling Presentation

The presentation is where recruiters evaluate how well candidates present themselves and communicate clinical data—essentially, how they would interact with the KOLs and HCPs in real life. It is an opportunity for you to showcase your knowledge of the pharmaceutical industry, your ability to communicate complex scientific information, and your skills in scientific presentation.

- *Understanding Your Audience:* Tailor your presentation to resonate with the hiring committee's specific interests and background. Research their therapeutic focus, challenges, and recent advancements to demonstrate your alignment with their goals.

- *Selecting an Appropriate Subject:* If you were not given any topic by the company, choose a topic that you are very confident and well-versed in. The topic you've chosen should also align with the company's interests and portfolio.

- *Crafting a Winning Structure:* Begin with a compelling introduction that immediately grabs the audience's interest and provides a concise overview of your main arguments or ideas. Use a structured approach to deliver information concisely, ending with a strong summary that reinforces your main arguments and leaves a lasting impression.

- *Showcasing Confidence in Delivery:* Project confidence through strong vocal tone, body language, and eye contact. Articulate your speech clearly, maintaining a steady pace while avoiding unnecessary filler words.

- *Injecting Storytelling in Narration:* Incorporate storytelling by framing your scientific paper or clinical data within a narrative structure, such as describing the journey of discovery or the evolution of understanding. Use anecdotes or case studies to humanize the data, illustrating its real-world impact or relevance. Engage your audience by emphasizing the challenges faced, the pivotal moments of insight, and the potential implications for healthcare or scientific advancement.

- *Using Visuals:* Employ visual aids such as images, graphs, and charts to illustrate key points, demonstrate experimental procedures, or showcase data trends. Ensure that your visuals are clear, relevant, and easy to understand. Take cues from how the KOLs present their work. You may be able to find their previous presentation online. Use their style and template, and if you're lucky, you may be able to download the PowerPoint template and use it. I followed this strategy, and I have heard many times that I was probably the most effective presenter in an interview.

- *Engaging Your Audience:* Encourage interaction by asking thought-provoking questions and inviting comments. Be prepared to handle unexpected inquiries with composure and analytical thinking. Like any good story, your scientific presentation should build tension and anticipation as you lead your audience through the research process. Highlight challenges, unanswered questions, or unexpected discoveries to keep your audience engaged. Avoid jargon and strive for clear and concise communication that everyone can understand.

- *Closing With Impact:* Summarize key points, reinforce your message, and end on a high note to leave a lasting impression.

- *Practice Makes Perfect:* Rehearse extensively to ensure smooth delivery, confident transitions, and precise timing. Familiarize yourself with the presentation software and troubleshoot technical issues beforehand.

Organizing the Presentation

The recruiters will either give you a topic for the presentation (usually a clinical paper the company published recently about a product) or allow for a topic of your choice. If it is the latter, it would be an amazing opportunity to showcase your expertise. Choose a topic that you are very confident and well-versed in. Also, the presentation should be tailored to the specific company and the role you are applying for.

Thorough preparation, confidence, and effective communication are essential for success in MSL presentations. Here's how you would want to outline your presentation:

Start with an introduction.

Your introduction should provide an overview of the clinical presentation and its purpose. You should also introduce yourself and your qualifications.

Present the background information.

In the next section of your presentation, you should provide background information on the topic that you are discussing. This could include information on the disease state, the clinical trial data, or the product that you are presenting. Also, discuss the current standard of care for this disease or condition and explain how this clinical paper is significant to address the issues with existing protocol.

Present the clinical data.

The main body of your presentation should focus on the clinical data. You should present the data in a clear and concise way, and you should highlight the key findings.

- **Methods:**
  - Describe the methods that were used in the clinical trial.
  - Discuss the study population and the inclusion/exclusion criteria.
  - Explain how the data was collected and analyzed.

- **Results:**
  - Present the key findings of the clinical trial.
  - Discuss the implications of these findings for the treatment of this disease or condition.

- **Discussion:**
  - Discuss the strengths and limitations of the clinical trial.
  - Identify areas for future research.

Discuss the implications for healthcare professionals.

The final section of your presentation should discuss the implications of the clinical data for healthcare professionals. You should discuss how the data can be used to improve patient care. Also, address the unmet need in the sector in light of the presentation. You can also highlight how the trial implicates the company strategy.

Create a cohesive ending to your presentation.

Your conclusion should summarize the key points of your presentation and restate the purpose of your presentation. You should also thank the audience for their time.

Questions to answer during the presentation.

The interviewer may ask you questions during your presentation. Be prepared to answer questions about the clinical data, the implications for healthcare professionals, or your qualifications.

Always keep in mind that all the candidates get the same instruction. It is up to you to separate yourself from the others and stand out. Always bring that level of interest and enthusiasm you felt when you saw the job opening to the interview room. A presentation is about telling a story and how well you connect the data to real-world medical practice. So, put a lot of effort and time into making your presentation compelling and interesting.

In addition to the content of your presentation, it is also important to consider the following factors:

- **Audience:** Who will be attending your presentation? What are their levels of expertise?

- **Delivery:** Speak clearly and concisely. Use visuals to help illustrate your points.

- **Engagement:** Ask the audience questions to keep them engaged.

Here are some tips for creating a successful interview presentation:

- Make sure that the clinical trial or the study you are using is recent and current.

- Do not turn the presentation into a data dump. There should be a balance of data and science in the presentation—it should be data-rich and scientifically rigorous enough for you to demonstrate your ability to convey scientific information effectively, accurately, and compellingly.

- Pay attention to details. Use a professional presentation software program, such as PowerPoint or Keynote.

- Use clear and concise fonts and graphics. Dark text like black or blue on a white background is always ideal. Do not use greens or yellows, as they could impact people with color blindness. Do not use a loud background.

- Do not over-complicate the presentation with unnecessary animation.

- Practice, practice, and practice.

- Be mindful of the time limit for your presentation. Generally, 15 minutes are assigned for a presentation. Prepare the right number of slides so you can go through them in the assigned timeframe, but remember that there's always going to be some variability depending on individuals and circumstances. Your goal is to tell your story within that timeframe. It is not an exam; rather, it is a measure of your understanding, preparedness, and communication skills.

- Always ask the hiring manager whether the assigned time would include the question/answer session and prepare accordingly.
- Don't forget to spellcheck your presentation!
- Lastly, be confident when delivering your presentation. **You got this!**

A Medical Science Liaison interview presentation is a valuable opportunity to showcase your skills and knowledge. By following the tips above, you can create a successful presentation that will impress the interviewers and increase your chances of landing the job.

Follow-up

Following the interview, it is advisable to create a personal summary encompassing the newly acquired information obtained during the interview. When taking notes, be sure to record your observations of the individuals you encountered, as well as specific information regarding the role and any other notable details that you can recall. While you may initially feel that you would retain all the information from your interviews, recollections tend to diminish over time. If you are applying for multiple opportunities or evaluating a few options, you will need to assess and pick the most suitable employment for you.

Compose an expression of gratitude promptly following the interview, ideally on the same day. It could be an email or a customized letter. Direct your address to the main interviewer while also acknowledging and mentioning the names of any individuals who provided particularly valuable assistance during the interview process. Maintain a positive tone in the note and utilize it to emphasize your ongoing enthusiasm for the position.

When being questioned by a group, it is advisable to send a thank you message to all individuals you interacted with, or at the absolute least, to the main interviewers. A thank-you note acts as an additional gesture that has the potential to distinguish oneself from another individual.

Reiterate the specific position you are applying for to the interviewer. Emphasize your enthusiasm for the role and the organization. Highlight one or two of your most powerful skills and customize them to address the needs of the interviewers.

Kindly provide your contact details along with the most convenient hours for contacting you. Conclude by proposing a recommendation for future action, such as arranging the next occasion for a meeting.

Keep your response in the note concise, limiting it to a maximum of 12 sentences. Eliminate any spelling errors, typographical mistakes, and other difficulties. Avoid giving the impression of either pleading or assuming that you already have the job.

Follow-up Email Format

Dear (Interviewer Name),

Thank you so much for taking the time to speak with me about the MSL position with [insert company name]. It was a pleasure to learn more about [insert commentary on discussion points or position information].

I am excited about the possibility of joining the team! The details of some of the projects we talked about are attached. Please feel free to contact me if you need any more information.

Thank you,
Your Name

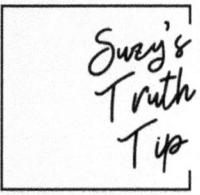

- *Stay up-to-date on the latest clinical research: The pharmaceutical industry is constantly evolving, so it's important to stay current on the latest clinical research. This will help you stay informed about new drugs and treatments, and it will also help you answer questions from healthcare professionals.*

- *Develop your communication skills: MSLs need to be able to communicate effectively with a variety of audiences, including healthcare professionals, patients, and the general public. Developing your communication skills will help you succeed in the role. Consider joining an organization like Toastmasters International to develop your public speaking skills.*

What NOT To Do: A Full Recap

When seeking a Medical Science Liaison (MSL) role, it is essential to distinguish oneself as a credible and knowledgeable applicant. Here are some things to avoid during your application process:

Avoid placing excessive emphasis on research experience at the expense of communication skills. As an MSL with a strong scientific foundation, you should demonstrate exceptional proficiency in converting intricate medical data into easily comprehensible information for healthcare providers, and you should also demonstrate your proficiency in communication. This includes abilities in delivering presentations, public speaking engagements, and written correspondence.

Never disregard the act of customizing your CV and cover letter. Tailor your materials to each unique job description, highlighting how your talents and expertise directly correspond with their specified requirements.

Do not underestimate the significance of networking. Contact MSLs that specialize in your field of interest or connect with alumni from your program. Networking can offer significant insights into the position, connect you with prospects, and demonstrate your drive.

Never exaggerate your accomplishments or credentials. Truthfulness and moral uprightness are of the utmost importance in the healthcare industry. Ensure that you provide an honest account of your experience and refrain from embellishing your talents or achievements.

Never disregard the importance of professionalism in your internet presence. Recruiters may review your social media accounts.

Ensure that your internet presence exhibits professionalism and is consistent with your career objectives.

Do not concentrate exclusively on the remuneration and perks. Although significant, pay should not be the exclusive motivating factor. Emphasize your fervor for the industry, aspiration to have a positive impact on patient results, and congruence with the company's objective.

Do not exhibit poor time management or communication skills. Respond to interview requests promptly, attend interviews punctually, and maintain clear and straightforward communication throughout the entire process.

Do not wear attire that is not suitable for the interview. Adhere to a professional and conservative dress code that aligns with the company's culture and the gravity of the position.

Never pose inconsequential or ill-prepared inquiries during the interview. Conduct thorough research on the organization and formulate well-thought-out inquiries pertaining to the MSL position and the distinct corporate culture.

Never exhibit negativity or express unfavorable opinions about former employers. Instead, direct your attention to the favorable components of your experience and how they prepare you for this fresh chance.

Is there room for salary negotiation when accepting an MSL position?

When accepting a job offer, it's essential to keep in mind that salary negotiation is always a possibility. Even in a highly specialized field like Medical Affairs, there is often room for discussion. By doing your homework, highlighting your unique skills and experience, and being clear and concise in your communication, you can make a strong case for increasing your salary. Remember that this is a two-way conversation, and your potential employer may be more willing to negotiate than you expect. Don't underestimate the value you bring to the table, and be confident in advocating for fair compensation.

Accepting the Offer

Congrats! You received the offer letter, and it's time for you to accept it. How do you proceed? First, **carefully review** if the terms outlined in the offer letter, including salary, benefits, or any additional clauses align with your expectations and requirements. Remember, if you are writing this to the Hiring Manager, use a **proper salutation**. **Express gratitude** for the opportunity and confirm your acceptance of the position. While it is important for the letter to be brief, it is also important to **clarify the terms** of employment in the letter. Also, mention the **date you are joining** the company. Additionally, consider any necessary **follow-up** steps and end the letter with a **professional sign-off**.

Utilize the format below and tailor it to suit your needs.

Subject: Acceptance of offer for the position of [position title]

Dear [Hiring Manager's Last Name],

I am writing to express my sincere gratitude for offering me the position at [company's name]. I have reviewed the terms of employment and am delighted to accept your offer.

As proposed, my annual salary will be [salary], and health and life insurance benefits will be provided for me and my family after 30 days of employment. I will officially begin my employment on [start date].

Please let me know if you require any further information or documentation. I look forward to completing all the remaining formalities prior to my joining, allowing for a smooth transition into my role.

Thank you again for this wonderful opportunity, and I look forward to working with you as a part of your team.

Yours sincerely,

[Your name/signature]

Request to be withdrawn from consideration for a position

So, you got the offer letter, but the terms of employment don't quite sit with you. Or, perhaps you have landed a better offer from a larger company. It could also be other reasons, i.e., personal issues, relocation, or compensation. Whatever the reason, it's crucial to *formally request withdrawal* from the position and to notify the employer right away. *Briefly explain* your reason for withdrawing while *maintaining a positive tone* to leave a good impression. I am sharing a sample below to help you:

Utilize the format below and tailor it to suit your needs.

Subject: Request to be withdrawn from a position

Dear [Hiring Manager's Last Name],

Thank you very much for considering me for the position of [position title] with [company name].

After careful consideration, I would like to withdraw my application for the role. This decision stems from [mention reasons, such as "accepting a position at another company," "relocation plans," "personal circumstances," "discrepancy in negotiated salary/terms of employment," etc.].

I sincerely appreciate you taking the time to interview me and to share information on the opportunity and your company. It was a pleasure meeting the team. Again, thank you for your consideration and the time you shared.

Sincerely,

[Your name/signature]

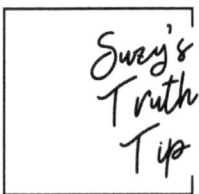

- *Do not be unprofessional*
- *Do not send more than one follow-up email inquiry or thank-you request*
- *Do not show up to someone's job*
- *Do not call to inquire what happened or advocate for yourself on the phone*
- *If you did not hear back, accept that you may not have gotten the job*

Afterword

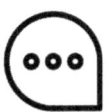

As you close this book, ready to embark on your exciting MSL journey, remember: the path may have twists and turns, but with dedication, passion, and the right guidance, you can navigate the maze and achieve your dream.

Believe in the power of your unique skill set. Combine your scientific depth with exceptional communication, unwavering curiosity, and a genuine desire to make a difference in patients' lives. This potent blend makes you an invaluable asset to the MSL community.

Remember, challenges are inevitable. Embrace them as opportunities to learn, grow, and refine your MSL expertise. Never shy away from asking questions, seeking mentorship, and collaborating with your peers. The MSL community is a supportive network, and I encourage you to actively engage and learn from its collective wisdom.

And finally, don't hesitate to reach out! Connect with me on LinkedIn (https://www.linkedin.com/in/suzannerabi) or follow me on social media (on TikTok, Instagram, or YouTube as @drsuzannesoliman). I'm passionate about empowering aspiring

MSLs and am always happy to offer guidance, share insights, and celebrate your successes.

This journey is yours to own. Embrace the challenges, celebrate the victories, and never lose sight of your passion for science and making a difference. Welcome to the MSL world, and remember, the maze may be intricate, but with perseverance and the right tools, you'll find your path to success.

With unwavering support,

Suzanne Soliman, PharmD, BCMAS

References

1. Kimble CA, Brazeau GA. Developing and Implementing a HyFlex Elective Course in Medical Affairs Addressing a Curricular Gap. *American Journal of Pharmaceutical Education*. 2023; 87(8):100290-100290. doi: https://doi.org/10.1016/j.ajpe.2023.100290

2. Kanmaz T, Mandler H, Soliman S, Rasty S. Are pharmacy schools adequately preparing graduates for roles in industry? Poster presented at the 119th Annual Meeting of the American Association of Colleges of Pharmacy, Boston, Massachusetts. *American Journal of Pharmaceutical Education*. 2018; 82(5):7158-7158. doi: https://doi.org/10.5688/ajpe7158

3. ACMA. Break into the MSL Role for the Right Reasons. medicalaffairsspecialist.org. Published May 11, 2021. Accessed March 15, 2024. https://medicalaffairsspecialist.org/blog/break-into-the-msl-role-for-the-right-reasons

4. Albert E, Sass C. *The Medical Science Liaison: An A to Z Guide*. Second Edition. Butler University Books; 2011. https://digitalcommons.butler.edu/butlerbooks/10

5. Medical Science Liaison Society. *USA Results 2022 MSL Salary & Compensation*; 2022. https://themsls.org/wp-content/uploads/2022/12/2022-Salary-Survey-_-USA.pdf

6. Yung A, Soliman SR. Medical science liaisons within the pharmaceutical industry: description and history. Poster presented at: 2019 American Society of Health-System Pharmacists. December 8-12, 2019; Las Vegas, Nevada. Published 2019. https://images.ctfassets.net/oovue9s2mk1n/1nudKvaZ-BOUooyReDzffw6/489560638160c8990c70ac951d13e14d/Midyear_Poster_11.30.19.pptx.png

7. U.S. BUREAU OF LABOR STATISTICS. Medical Scientists: Occupational Outlook Handbook: U.S. Bureau of Labor Statistics. Bls.gov. Published October 23, 2018. https://www.bls.gov/ooh/life-physical-and-social-science/medical-scientists.htm

8. Soliman W. Pharma's Navy Seals: The Medical Science Liaison. www.linkedin.com. Published September 15, 2019. Accessed March 19, 2024. https://www.linkedin.com/pulse/pharmas-navy-seals-medical-science-liaison-soliman-phd-bcmas-/?trk=article-ssr-frontend-pulse_more-articles_related-content-card

9. ACMA. *Medical Affairs Essentials: Career Options for Medical Science Liaisons*; Published August 9, 2021. Accessed April 1, 2024. https://medicalaffairsspecialist.org/blog/msl-alternatives

10. Van Zee A. The Promotion and Marketing of OxyContin: Commercial Triumph, Public Health Tragedy. *American Journal of Public Health*. 2009;99(2):221-227. doi: https://doi.org/10.2105/ajph.2007.131714

11. Rutherford P, Smith N. *Medical Science Liaisons: A Key to Driving Patient Access to New Therapies*; 2016. https://www.iqvia.com/-/media/library/white-papers/medical-science-liaisons.pdf

12. Medical Science Liaison: What Comes Next in the Career? | IQVIA news and blogs. IQVIA. Published November 2022. Accessed March 20, 2024. https://www.iqviamedicalsalescareers.com/article/2022-11/what-is-the-next-step-after-medical-science-liaison

13. Dixson K. How Much Do MSLs Make? Medical Science Liaison Salary Insights. medicalaffairsspecialist.org. Published December 13, 2023. Accessed March 18, 2024. https://medicalaffairsspecialist.org/blog/medical-science-liaisons-salary

14. *2022 Job Seeker Nation Report*. https://web.jobvite.com/rs/328-BQS-080/images/2022-12-2022JobSeekerNationReport.pdf

15. Hu J. Over 98% of Fortune 500 Companies Use Applicant Tracking Systems (ATS) - Jobscan Blog. Published June 20, 2018. https://www.jobscan.co/blog/fortune-500-use-applicant-tracking-systems/

16. Caravela T. Resume Writing and Editing Tips for Pharma Professionals. Accreditation Council for Medical Affairs. Published August 2, 2019. Accessed March 22, 2024. https://old.medicalaffairsspecialist.org/resume-writing-and-editing-tips-for-pharma-professionals/

17. Resume Genius. 50+ Cover Letter Statistics for 2023 (Hiring Manager Survey). resumegenius.com. Published May 14, 2023.

https://resumegenius.com/blog/cover-letter-help/cover-letter-statistics

18. Medical Science Liaison Job Titles. SEMbio. Accessed March 24, 2024. https://sembiogroup.com/medical-science-liaison-job-titles/

19. Dahl K. Setting Your Course to a Successful MSL Career. Published March 16, 2020. Accessed March 25, 2024. https://medicalaffairsspecialist.org/blog/setting-your-course-to-successful-msl-career

20. ACMA. Specialized Certificate Programs. Accessed March 25, 2024. https://medicalaffairsspecialist.org/certificate-programs

21. ACMA. Science Behind the Magic. Accessed March 25, 2024. https://www.medicalaffairsspecialist.org/resources/acma-research#:~:text=87%25%20of%20KOLs%20surveyed%20(n

22. ACMA. Requiring BCMAS for Medical Science Liaison and Medical Affairs Roles. Published August 1, 2023. Accessed March 25, 2024. https://medicalaffairsspecialist.org/blog/board-certification-for-ma-and-msl

23. Dixon K. A Guide to Becoming a MSL. medicalaffairsspecialist.org. Published December 23, 2021. Accessed March 25, 2024. https://medicalaffairsspecialist.org/blog/guide-to-becoming-a-msl

24. Alexander J, Bunkers L, Dodd L, et al. *Analysis of 2020-2021 PharmD Industry Fellowships.*

REFERENCES

The following graphics used in this book all come from thenounproject.com collection:

- "timeline" by David Christensen in Chapter 1
- "job" by adi_sena in Chapter 2
- "roadmap" by Chimol in Chapter 3
- "Social Media" by Sunardi in Chapter 4
- "CV" by Distrologo in Chapter 5
- "cover letter" by annisa luthfiasari in Chapter 6
- "Job Search" by parnowowo in Chapter 7
- "Certificate" by Colourcreatype in Chapter 8
- "interview" by Alzam in Chapter 9
- "questions" by Seochan in Chapter 10
- "presentation" by Bahrul Ulum in Chapter 11
- "thought cloud" by Doodle Icons in Afterword

About the Author

Dr. Suzanne Soliman earned her PharmD from the University of Illinois at Chicago College of Pharmacy. She completed an education-focused primary care residency at Midwestern University Chicago College of Pharmacy and a teaching fellowship at UIC College of Medicine. She is a board-certified medical affairs specialist (BCMAS). Suzy was a clinical pharmacist, medical science liaison, and national field team instructor before becoming UIC-COP's Assistant Dean of Academic Affairs. Most recently, she was Associate Dean at Touro College of Pharmacy New York and independent pharmacy owner. Currently, she serves as ACMA's Chief Medical Officer.

In 2017, Suzy demonstrated her leadership skills by founding the largest US pharmacist group, Pharmacist Moms Group, which now boasts over 45,000 members. Her influence extends beyond this group, as she is a sought-after speaker nationwide on pharmacy, parenting, and women's issues. Her expertise is also evident in her extensive publication record, with over 100 publications to her name. Suzy's contributions have been recognized with prestigious awards, including the Next Generation Pharmacist Civic Leader Award, the Rufus A. Lyman Award for the best American Journal of Pharmacy Education paper, and the New Jersey Pharmacists Association Pharmaceutical Industry Award in 2021.

Suzy is a medical specialist and journal reviewer for *Annals of Pharmacotherapy* and *Currents in Pharmacy Teaching and Learning*. *The New York Times*, ABC7NY, *Daily Voice*, *New York Magazine*, *Crain's Chicago Business*, *Time Out Chicago*, and others have featured her. Suzy loves spending time with her husband and children, cooking, baking, and eating.

www.ingramcontent.com/pod-product-compliance
Lightning Source LLC
Chambersburg PA
CBHW051205120626
46547CB00013B/1215